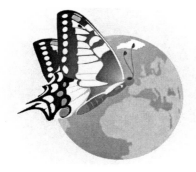

JOSHUA'S LESSONS

Raising a Healthy Child in a Toxic World

Published in the United States by Booklocker.com, Inc. Bangor, Maine.

The author of this book does not dispense medical advice nor prescribe the use of any technique as a form of treatment for physical or medical problems. The intent of the author is to offer information of a general nature to help in the quest to heal your self. The author assumes no responsibility in the event you use any of the information in this book for yourself or your family.

Printed in the United States of America on acid-free paper.

http://healingyou.com/
info@healingyou.com

JOSHUA'S LESSONS

Raising a Healthy Child in a Toxic World

Linda Wojcik

Dedication

To my son, Joshua, who taught me some of the most important lessons life has to offer. Thank you for choosing me to help guide you along life's magical pathways.

To my two daughters, Shannon and Holly Beth, whose love and support helped me devote the time and energy needed to help their brother heal.

Together, you are a light to the world.

Acknowledgements

I would like to acknowledge my brother, Gary Gallucci, who devoted countless hours editing Joshua's Lessons and through his encouraging thoughts and words helped me to achieve the strength and confidence to share Joshua's story with you.

I must also acknowledge Dr. William Shevin, who may have often thought me crazy but was kind enough never to say it out loud. Your insights and guidance helped me learn more about alternative therapies which in turn helped Joshua heal. Joshua's constitutional remedy was one of his saving graces both then and now.

Table of Contents

Foreword by Joshua's Sisters

My name is Shannon Kashmann and I am Joshua's older sister.

When I was growing up, all I wanted to do was fit in, avoid attention, and get on with life. With my brother's chemical sensitivities, trying to achieve any of these goals was nearly impossible. When my parents decided to go the "all-natural, organic" route, I didn't think much of it. As a seven year old, my thought was, "What does food really matter to me?" How little I knew.

Let me paint an image for you. You sit down at lunch surrounded by other children all eagerly tearing open their brown paper lunch bags or plopping down their hot lunch trays while you sit quietly with your Tupperware lunch container. You dread opening it; you know nothing "normal" is inside. There are no Twinkies, no white bread sandwiches, no Doritos. Instead, there is a wheat bread sandwich and BLUE corn chips! Oh and it's 1986, blue chips and wheat bread are NOT considered "cool!"

At times, I looked at Joshua in disgust, "How could you do this to me?" Then I'd remember the days and nights when he would throw himself on the floor, knocking his head against hard wood. I remember how the changes in our diets changed him for the better. In the end, the "sacrifices" I made, bringing un-cool food to school, were worth watching him get healthy.

As I look back now, I know that we all had to make sacrifices both for him and the family. After adjusting to our new eating lifestyle and realizing it wasn't so bad, I sat back and watched my brother transform. He went from this out of control child to a person who could communicate effectively with others; he was able to take criticisms and the word "NO" without losing his mind. It all started to make sense. The changes we were making in our lives were working for him.

My most treasured memory of my brother was when he stood up to the school board to convince them that the poisons on the school fields were harming not only him, but everyone. It still amazes me how powerful he was. His one voice woke up a small town and they stopped spraying pesticides. He wasn't afraid to show people who he was or what this world was doing to him. He stood there and let them all see him for him. How many of us can say that?

Last year at my brother's wedding, his two best men and lifelong friends, stood up to give their speeches. They each took a turn to talk about the man my brother had become, who he had been, and what he meant to them. We laughed about the days when he had to pack food to leave home, when a cell phone made him dizzy, and new clothing had to be washed prior to wearing. Listening to their stories, I turned to my mom and said, "Josh could have been the geek at school who everyone bullied. Instead, he was an amazing kid who knew what bothered him and was not afraid to express it." He was never afraid to tell his friends he needed "special care."

In the end, my brother was a popular member of the basketball team and the all-around good guy. Why? Because he knew what made him feel bad and what didn't, and he worked relentlessly with my mom to make changes in our community and in our lives.

Today, my brother doesn't need as much special care; however, he is cautious about what he puts into his body, knowing what it has done in the past and could easily do again. I now have a son of my own who, though not as sensitive as my little bro, has his own issues. I take special care to make sure he gets the best of everything especially the food and water we put into his body. I know from experience that what you eat affects who you are. I want my son to have the best life he can, without labels or judgments, just like his Uncle Josh.

My name is Holly Beth Corbin and I am Joshua's little sister.

Me: "I have the worst headache!"

World: "I have Advil…"

Me: "I have NEVER taken an Advil in my whole life."

World: (GASP)

Me: "AND…I'm not even immunized!"

World: (Double GASP!!) Looks of disgust are shot my way, shock, fear. These are the same people I have worked with for three years. Well, let me tell you about my brother.

Joshua was a chemically sensitive child; he was given many special treatments to stay healthy. He was allergic to EVERYTHING! When I came along, three years later, it was assumed I may be just as sensitive so I was treated as he was. No shots, no children's Tylenol, no chemicals in any food or cleaning supplies, only homeopathy and natural food.

My nickname throughout school was "Little Woj," and that was always a name I was proud of. Although, I have to admit, being Joshua Wojcik's little sister wasn't cool until high school; Josh was a tough act to follow.

Let's start with the water…when I was five, my sensitive brother had already learned the school water made him sick. I remember going into my kindergarten class with my water bottle and a note for the teacher. Every morning we formed a line in front of the teacher's desk if we had special notes or instructions. I was excited to have special instructions! I was to only drink from this water bottle, no water fountain for this girl! How exciting! My teacher rolled her eyes, no big deal to her, but it was very clear she did not care or want to understand what message this five year old was giving anyone.

I was always proud to be different. Maybe because my brother was so graceful and strong about what he would eat and wouldn't eat. I followed him wherever he went and wanted to be just like him.

I remember the smell of paint making him sick. In seventh grade, my school painted the gym floor. A few days later, gym class was held in that same enclosed gym area; did it reek of fumes! Am I the only one with a nose? My brother would have surely died! The next day I proudly marched up to my gym teacher and showed her my note from my mom.

She had the same reaction as my kindergarten teacher; eye roll followed by a definite sigh, "Well I don't know what good this is going to do you, Wojcik. You're going to have to sit out gym, IN THE GYM." She was angry at me. I never understood why people got mad. Did people get mad at my brother? I looked up to him. He had a message for everyone and no one cared to listen. Well, that made me mad! I sat in the gym and pondered, all the while getting a massive headache. Thanks, gym teacher!

I'll never forget when I was in eighth grade and my brother was getting sick in high school because they sprayed the football fields with pesticides. He had to get a tutor because he could not go near the school. It was strange to me that he was being schooled at home away from his friends. I'd just die! I felt sad for him, but he taught me that you should do anything for your health, even if it means sacrificing your social life for a few months.

My brother paved the way for me in school. I will always owe him for that. I may have been the annoying kid to teachers in middle school because I had semi-special needs. But in high school, I was never looked at as the "chemically sensitive kid's little sister." I was "Little Woj." Leave it to my brother to make it cool to be allergic to everything.

He made my life better. He was the guinea pig, the source for trial and error for what would make him sick and what was okay. I never had to drink the chlorine water from the water fountain. The fields at the high school were changed to organic fertilizer, and I never got sick from them. If I smelled paint in the hall, I knew to tell my mom. He taught me how to protect myself. He also taught me how to pay attention to what I was feeling and find the origins of it. Most importantly, he taught me that it was okay to be different.

We know what makes us sick, and we will avoid it at all costs, even if we get an eye roll here and there. I always wanted to be like my older brother, not in the "I'm allergic to everything" way, but in the "I will do what it takes to be healthy" way.

Introduction

Children who are born into the world today have in their possession an inherent knowledge and clear-cut responsibility at the time of their birth. They have accepted the challenge to heal our planet. These sensitive beings instinctively perceive a problem that needs immediate attention. It is our responsibility, as their parents, to guide and support their actions.

Joshua is my son, and this is his story. From the moment of his birth, I realized he was on an important mission. It would take years to understand the extent of his mission and the effects it would have on the entire community.

His journey began with a unique language that was often misunderstood, not only by those around him, but by both of us as well. It became my full time job to help Joshua interpret the meaning behind his symptoms.

Joshua was often on a physical and emotional roller coaster ride. His symptoms and reactions resembled those of children who were being diagnosed with ADD, ADHD, and ODD. However, medical labels and drug therapies were never part of Joshua's healing plan. We took a route considered extremely unorthodox and revolutionary for its time. Food became our medicine and alternative therapies replaced health insurance.

Joshua's bouts of anger and fear, of rage and crying forced me to look at possible causes that to my knowledge had not previously been explored. I introduced organic food, homeopathic medicines and natural products into our lives with the intent of keeping my son free of allopathic medicines and medical labels. I cleaned up our environment, cabinets, and refrigerator. With each change, Joshua began to heal.

Over time I came to understand he had a mission to help create a world free of chemicals and toxins. To accomplish this task, he had to initiate change in a world where change is often resisted. I wholeheartedly supported his efforts and subsequently shared what I learned from Joshua with everyone who was willing to listen.

Joshua was safe and healthy at home. Beyond those boundaries lingered a very different world. As he grew and ventured further from home, it became evident that he and I had to work together to initiate change throughout our community. Creating a safe space at school was our greatest challenge. We were confronted with many obstacles from those who had the power to help him heal. He needed compassion and understanding; he received intolerance and fear.

By nature, the human condition rejects change. More often than not, Joshua's mission was met with profound resistance. Fortunately, resistance seemed to hold no power over him. He learned to face his fears, and in turn, was the encouraging force to help those in authority face their own fears.

By the simple act of reading his story, you will learn a new and exciting language. It is a language of the human spirit; a language that requires immediate love and attention. Our sensitive children elicit hope for the future by demanding radical changes in the present. We have little time to waste.

This next generation has been tasked with charting our future course as human beings. We are required to act now to provide our children the opportunity to live in a world that is free of chemicals, fear, and anger. In so doing, we can help create peace and spiritual joy on a planet that will no longer accept anything else.

Joshua's story is about one young boy who took on the establishment for his right to be healthy at home and at school. To do that, he had to come up against his greatest rivalry, chemicals known as pesticides. More often than not, the pesticides won. In the end, however, Joshua learned many valuable lessons about healing chemical sensitivities in a chemically influenced world. We are happy to share them all with you. These are Joshua's lessons.

Joshua's Lessons

- Pure water is essential
- Avoid chemicals in my food, water and environment
- Milk is not good for everyone
- Not all corn muffins are created equal
- Be patient, healing takes time and energy
- Read every label
- Discipline is a necessity
- No one knows more about Joshua than Joshua
- Truth is the same as love
- There is a solution to every problem
- Diplomacy helps create peace
- Be responsible for healing myself
- Honor my needs
- Choose supportive friends
- Stand strong in my beliefs
- Emotions create physical symptoms
- Be accountable for my own thoughts, words and actions
- Love all of myself, even my sensitive nature
- Forgive others; they just don't know
- Healing occurs within

Chapter One

~ Joshua's Mission ~

Joshua was born on a cold January morning in 1982. He was the second of three children, my first and only son. He came to me both chemically sensitive and dairy allergic. I am certain that was not by chance. Both conditions forced me to devote much of my time helping my son heal these imbalances. There was much to learn.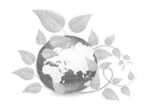

There is a great deal more to Joshua's story than a single child in need of healing. Joshua was charged with a knowing that came from deep within himself; a charge to protect himself and the environment in which he lived. It was a mission he was not allowed to dismiss. It would take years to accomplish this mission; he learned patience.

Joshua was constantly demanding my attention through a language that many were incapable of understanding. The language manifested as physical symptoms and emotional imbalances. I learned his language by paying attention and listening intently to what he was trying to convey.

His two sisters, Shannon and Holly Beth, were both compassionate toward their brother's needs. This assured me the time necessary to help their brother heal. To this day, they periodically see fit to remind me that Joshua has always been my favorite. My counter argument is that he just needed me more.

The truth is that Joshua was a single child armed with the power to change the course of many lives. Over time, it became evident that Joshua's experiences would initiate change throughout the entire community. His lessons influenced a great number of people who are now conscious about the foods they eat, the water they drink and the environment in which they live.

Before any of this came to pass, Joshua had to learn what caused his own imbalances and then to share that knowledge with me. We learned together. For years we watched, we listened, we talked and we shared. Challenges arose; we met each one. Problems occurred; we found solutions. As time went on, Joshua's most important lesson of all was very simple and, just like Joshua, very profound: *healing occurs within.*

It took Joshua a long time to learn that lesson, and the years following up to it caused Joshua a great deal of physical and emotional pain. When he finally recognized the pain as an opportunity to heal, he was able to move beyond it. Beyond the pain he embraced truth, compassion and understanding, three energies that stimulated his ability to heal.

Joshua is not the only child born to help heal the earth; he is far from alone. He arrived early to pave the way for those who would follow, and if by chance you have been guided to read his story, it may be because you are being divinely directed to learn about your own sensitive child.

There are many souls who have since come to finish what Joshua began. They are being diagnosed with ADD and ADHD, Autism and behavioral problems. None of these labels describe who they are, sensitive beings with a mission to change the world. To accomplish their goals, they have to speak loud and clear. They are screaming to be heard. It is time for all of us to listen.

Tender Loving Care

When Joshua was only six months old, my husband Ken and I opened our first health food store in Connecticut. There would be many more to follow. Opening our store at that particular time was a conscious choice that would allow us to learn alternative ways to help our son heal his dairy allergies and chemical sensitivities. In the not so distant future, our little store would become a haven for those searching to avoid dairy products as well as chemicals in their food, water and environment. Joshua was the enlightening force toward a healthy lifestyle.

We recognized Joshua's allergy to milk and his sensitivities to various chemicals at a very young age. Through the years, we learned how to deal with each threat to his health individually. While it was overwhelming and frustrating at times, I eventually realized Joshua's sensitive nature was a gift for the entire family.

At first, however, it was far more of a challenge, as I was attempting to raise a chemically sensitive child in a chemically influenced world. Over time we learned that for every problem we faced, there was a solution to be found. We worked endlessly to find each one. Joshua soon learned the art of problem solving.

With Joshua's help, I realized that chemically sensitive children can live normal, healthy lives in spite of the inhibitions presented by the world surrounding them. All they need is tender loving care from a supportive family and a safe haven in which to heal. Our chemical free home was Joshua's safe haven.

Sensitive children also need the people they associate with on a daily basis to respect their special needs and requirements. Our greatest challenge was to persuade those in authority to change their behaviors to accommodate one very special child. Not everyone was easily persuaded.

There are potentially numerous situations that might occur each day around our neighborhoods, in our schools and on our playing fields that can turn a perfectly healthy child into a very ill child within a matter of moments. Joshua and I worked adamantly to change the habits of our community and schools for his right to be healthy.

Mastering the Art of Healing

During his high school years, both the school and its surrounding fields became so toxic to Joshua's system that he was unable to be in or around the school. Most of the latter portion of his junior year was spent with a tutor at home. More than anything else, Joshua wanted those in power to respect his right to an education. His heart was telling him he needed to be at school; his body was telling him school had become a "playground of poisons." His thoughts were in constant emotional turmoil. The toxic fields won.

It was during this time that I recognized a clear pattern of behavior; or, in this case, a clear pattern of reaction. The more frustrated Joshua became with the situation at school, the faster and more intensely his body reacted.

Thoughts are energy, and energy is a creative force. Every creative force needs direction. How we choose to direct each thought is consistent to what we are creating in our lives. For instance, a negative thought has the power to create a negative outcome; a positive thought has the power to create a positive outcome. To heal, Joshua had to recognize how he was powering his own thoughts. Once recognized he had an opportunity to change them; one thought at a time.

While I shared these observations with my son, it was up to him to recognize them, to embrace them, and to do everything possible to try to change his own behaviors. The ensuing journey seemed long and arduous at times, but in the end rewards were reaped. Joshua was mastering the art of healing himself.

This played a huge role in allowing him to become a leader and a teacher in the community. As with every great teacher, his teachings were not easily accepted by those in authority. Yet that never hampered his efforts; it only made him stronger in his beliefs and in his mission.

Joshua understood that there are many paths to healing. The more paths we experience, the more we learn about ourselves. The more we learn, the more we understand what makes our bodies happy and what does not. Joshua learned to focus on what did.

The food we eat and the water we drink can also help us heal. Food and water have the potential to nourish our bodies or, conversely, to feed our pains. The question remains, why can some people eat chemically altered food day in and day out and appear unaffected? Why are some of us sensitive, while others are not? There are answers to these questions, and Joshua provided the doorway to those answers.

Chapter Two

~ Dairy Allergies ~

Long before we thought about chemical sensitivities, we realized that Joshua had dairy allergies. Back in the early 80s dairy allergies were not as accepted or understood as they are today. What I learned about dairy allergies came through Joshua. He was my teacher.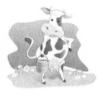

When Joshua was three months old, I was no longer able to nurse him. Life got in the way as it often does. I wanted to avoid putting him on baby formula; I was hoping to find something more natural. I remembered a story my Italian grandmother shared with me after my first baby was born:

The last children my grandmother birthed were a set of twins. She did not have enough milk to nurse both babies and turned to raw cow milk to help supplement her own. Because money was tight, my grandfather purchased a family cow. Both babies did well on raw cow's milk. She was happy with her choice.

Now that I was having the same dilemma with my own baby, that memory reappeared. However, I realized that milk from a family cow was far different from milk on our grocery shelves. I felt a better choice would be organic cow's milk. I drove to the nearest health food store and purchased Joshua's first bottle. It did not take long to realize I was not going to be quite as happy with my choice as my grandmother was with hers.

It was a beautiful spring day and friends had come to visit. The children were playing in the fields behind our home. Diane and I enjoyed watching their antics. I filled Joshua's bottle with organic cow milk and began feeding him. He liked it; his body did not. Within minutes, he was covered in a rash from head to toe. I was examining my baby when Diane asked, "Why are you not taking this child to the nearest hospital?"

I suppose any other mother would have done just that, however, I was not any other mother. Diane was surprised by my answer, "This is the first time I gave him cow's milk and he immediately broke out in a rash. Instead of rushing him to a hospital, I think I will stop the cow's milk and see if the rash disappears." I thought that was a good idea. I did not fancy hospitals, and the thought of them poking and prodding my baby for a rash that might have a known cause made me feel uncomfortable. The rash slowly disappeared on its own.

That was my first realization that if I put something new into Joshua's young body, he might experience a reaction; he was obviously having a reaction to the milk. My next thought was "What would I do instead? I did not want to rely on formula.

The Alternative to Cow's Milk

Since our first child 4 years previously, I had become an avid student of natural foods and holistic medicines. I read every book available at the time. Food having the potential to cause allergic reactions was a subject that was familiar to me. I was not shocked that a little body might react to cow's milk. Many people it seems reacted to cow's milk.

Through my studies, I learned that goat's milk could be the perfect alternative for those who were allergic to cow's milk, especially young children. My thoughts immediately turned toward that direction.

We were fortunate to live in a very rural area surrounded by a vast array of small local farms. It did not take long to search out the nearest goat milk farm. I purchased Joshua's first quart of goat's milk that day. Realizing the richness of goat milk, I cut it in half with pure spring water. Joshua loved it. I waited for a reaction; any reaction. He had none. His body was happy and so was I. My long thin baby quickly began to gain the few extra pounds he needed.

I treated this modification seriously. I researched goat's milk before introducing it 100% into his diet. In my research I learned that goat's milk is much like mother's milk except it is deficient in folic acid. We've all come to learn the importance of folic acid in our diets, especially for young babies. Obviously it's not as important for baby goats. Since Joshua's main staple was to be goat's milk, a folic acid deficiency would be a huge problem. To solve the problem, I ordered a folic acid capsule. Each morning, I broke the capsule open and put a little of the folic acid powder on my wet finger. Then I put the vitamin directly on Joshua's tongue; he liked it.

This adjustment to Joshua's diet was made without informing his pediatrician. I had a tendency to do things like that. I knew Joshua's next baby visit would be the moment of truth. I would have to share this information with his doctor.

Although I felt confident in my decision, I did feel a bit apprehensive about sharing this information after the fact. However, no one could deny that Joshua was content, happy and healthy. The good fat in goat milk was helping him gain the few extra pounds he desperately needed. I was hopeful that his pediatrician agreed with me.

Informing the Doctor

The pediatrician I had at the time was not holistic, but he was flexible and open minded. We had an honest relationship. He knew I was very different from most moms, and he respected most of my decisions without question.

I could feel my anxiety increase as I entered his office. I took a seat across from him; Joshua sat in my lap. With a little fear in my voice, I began to share my story. He listened to my concerns about baby formulas, Joshua's reaction to organic cow milk and finally my choice to try goat milk. He showed no emotion; he simply allowed me to talk. When I finally finished, he sat back and said, "Are you aware that goat's milk is deficient in folic acid?" I was impressed he knew.

"Yes, I am aware. I researched goat's milk before I gave it to Josh. I solved that problem by buying a folic acid capsule. I put a little on his tongue every day." I could tell he was impressed that I did my research, and he could not deny that Joshua's overall physical appearance had improved. By the time our visit was over, he felt comfortable with my decision. He blessed Joshua's new diet.

Eliminate the Problem

At first goat milk was used only for Joshua. It was expensive and he was the one who needed it most. So we continued to have milk and milk products in the house for everyone else. As Joshua got older, this did not turn out to be such a good idea. Having these products in the house was a temptation to all of us. It became easy to give him just a little of this or a little of that. On a positive note, those little bits of "this and that" allowed me to recognize different symptoms from different products.

Over time I realized that Joshua's sensitivity to cow milk products was extreme. Even small amounts of milk produced symptoms that ranged from a simple runny nose to an all-out asthma attack. Whenever we allowed Joshua to cheat with just a little, there was ALWAYS a reaction, some major, many minor. Each reaction was another lesson in healing.

Eventually, I realized it was not healthy to have cow's milk in the house at all. Small amounts in food or drink had the potential to set off a reaction that could last for days. It was not worth the risks. Nor was it healthy for us to eat food he was allergic to in front of him. Our support was becoming essential.

One day I decided it was time to clean out the refrigerator. Anything that remotely resembled milk on the label was discarded. I had enough experience with him by then to know that just a little milk was probably too much. If you want to completely clean out a body, you have to completely eliminate the problem; and cow dairy was a problem.

Our family became cow dairy-free that day. Our cupboards were filled with soy this and rice that. Finding new products that contained goat milk was an exciting event, especially if it tasted good!

Soon thereafter, I realized something amazing. Eliminating milk from our diets greatly improved all our health. My husband stopped continuously clearing his throat, Shannon's chronic cough improved and my skin cleared up. Who would have known?

How Much Is Too Much?

Owning a health food store proved valuable. Joshua liked to eat and he needed food that was pure. It also had to taste good in order for him to eat it. I filled the shelves with products taste tested by Joshua. Like every child, snacks were important; it was equally important they were free of all cow dairy.

Joshua was my partner at our health food store and cafe. I loved working with him. By the time he turned two, I gave him jobs to do to keep him busy throughout the day. He rearranged the shelves; and at the end of the day I arranged them back. We were both proficient at our jobs!

Payment at the end of each work day was important. We designed a payment option that suited both our needs. Joshua was allowed to choose one small snack at the end of each day. As I cashed out the register, Joshua scoured the shelves. Candy was rare at home, so naturally it was his first choice to serve as his paycheck for a hard day's work. I allowed him that option.

His dairy allergies limited his candy choices. Most chocolate was full of dairy. That would not do, and I didn't particularly like feeding caffeine to his sensitive body either.

Carob was an alternative that we explored. Some of it was very tasty; much was not. We tried to fill the shelves with carob that was approved by Joshua's taste buds. His favorite was a little nickel size carob candy with mint flavoring.

When this new treat entered the store, it immediately became his "payment of choice." We performed our payment ritual each evening. With a smile on his face, Joshua held out his hand in anticipation of his nightly treat. I was happy to oblige. He immediately devoured it. A long day's work for a moment of pleasure! The size of the treat had no meaning to Joshua. It was the taste that mattered.

It was not long after the carob introduction that Joshua developed a constant sniffle. Between fixing Joshua's shelving projects, I spent the rest of my day grabbing tissues to wipe his runny nose. He didn't like it, and neither did I.

One day as we were getting ready to close the shop, a friend stopped by on her way home from work. She waited patiently while Joshua ate his daily ration and I wiped his nose. Kathy was very aware of Joshua's sensitivities. She commented as he eagerly opened the wrapper, "Do you think that candy might contain dairy?" I was faced with my own denial.

I was embarrassed to admit that I had not read the package label. After all, how much damage could one small piece of candy cause? I picked up the package and to my not-so-surprise, the third ingredient on the list was "milk." Why hadn't I thought of that myself? My moment of guilt quickly passed as I dealt with the situation.

I sat down with Joshua and explained, "I think this candy is causing your runny nose. I think if we found a different snack that did not contain milk, you might feel better. Are you willing to stop eating it for a little while and see what happens?"

As little as he was, Joshua understood clearly. He did not like being sick. He liked feeling healthy. He stopped eating his favorite candy. We promptly found a replacement that was free of any cow dairy ingredients. I read the label before offering it to him.

It did not take long to notice a difference. Within a few days, Joshua's runny nose completely disappeared. It was a huge lesson for both of us. Avoiding all cow dairy was important for Joshua's health. Just a little was way too much!

Joshua was teaching us how food affected all of us. His body spoke loud and clear; our bodies were not as outspoken. The entire family was beginning to understand that food is much like medicine. It can nourish and heal; it also has the potential to cause physical symptoms.

I liked the lessons we were learning together. Joshua was learning that he was in charge of his healing; I was learning not to force my will upon him. Instead I encouraged him to make healthy choices, and I watched as he consciously chose to be healthy.

Yes, We Have No Cow's Milk

As long as we were strict and dairy free, Joshua was free of symptoms. I learned to read labels and eliminated all food that contained whey and nonfat dry milk, along with anything else that remotely resembled cow's milk. In the real world, however, it was more difficult to keep him away from cow dairy. Although I tried to educate our family and friends, no one wanted to believe that milk could have such a damaging effect on a person. After all, isn't milk good for everyone? The truth was milk was not good for Joshua.

My family and many of our friends thought we were being too strict. How could anyone live without milk? Often they encouraged Joshua to eat something he knew he should avoid. This was not easy for him. He was afraid of upsetting the adults who thought they knew better.

I struggled to convince everyone that their offerings were detrimental to Joshua's health; however, they had their own thoughts and ideas of what Joshua could and should be eating. Often, they served him food they knowingly contained dairy.

Although their intentions were good, even small amounts of milk could undermine all his work. In the end it was he and I who suffered the consequences for their actions. Joshua would end up sick and sometimes it took days to recover.

Finally, I stopped trying to persuade them; I insisted. I was his mother and I had the final word in what he ate. I let everyone know my feelings. With my persistence, everyone finally adjusted to Joshua's lack of milk in his diet.

I learned, however, that if I wanted others to respect our choices, I had to learn to respect theirs as well. So I picked my battles carefully. When my mother visited, she brought her own coffee, sugar and milk. I poured myself a cup of Kaffree Roma, pure maple syrup and soy milk. We were learning to laugh about our differences instead of fighting over them. What other people consumed was not my concern, nor did it affect me. I liked our new way of eating and so did Joshua.

Symptoms of Dairy Allergies

Joshua lived comfortably on goat's milk. Eventually, soy and rice products were introduced. Each time I introduced something new I paid attention to his body. If it wasn't good for him, I knew almost instantly! He was like a little computer, giving me positive or negative responses depending upon if his body was happy or not.

As time went on, the original rash no longer plagued him; his body responded to dairy with sinus and breathing problems. The severity of the symptoms was also dependent upon how much dairy was in the product he consumed. I learned to pay close attention to his reactions whenever anyone gave him something with dairy in it. Most of the time his nose would run, but if the food contained too much dairy, his lungs were affected. Feeling like he could not get enough air into his lungs was devastating. His life simply came to a standstill.

Over time, Joshua revealed many physical symptoms that were associated with his sensitivity to cow milk products. These symptoms included: *Digestive problems, skin rashes, acne, sinus infections, abdominal cramping, bronchial infections, ear infections and asthma.*

Dairy Allergies and School

Convincing family and friends that milk is not good for everyone is one thing. Convincing a school system is another.

Joshua turned five years old in January of 1987. Until this time, he lived in the safety of our home. We knew this could not last forever. The day came when Joshua needed to leave his safe haven and enter the world of classrooms and teachers.

That was a scary day for all of us. At home or at the store, we controlled what he ate and what entered his environment. We had to prepare him for the outside world. We talked extensively of the things he needed to do for himself.

Milk allergies were not common in the late 80s when Joshua entered school. The school system did not know what to make of him. Milk is a staple for the school lunch program. Everyone had to have it; everyone except Joshua.

He had to be prepared to teach the teachers what he could and could not have. What I didn't realize was how hard it was going to be and how long it was going to take.

The summer before Joshua started Kindergarten, I made an appointment with the school principal to inform her of Joshua's dairy allergies. I also informed her that I would provide snacks and drinks for Joshua and that the school was not to feed him anything.

"I am afraid, Mrs. Wojcik, that we cannot comply with your request without an official note from a doctor."

"Why?" I asked. "What did a doctor have to do with my son's allergies? When did I, as his mother, give up my right to decide what my child consumes? I am the one who feeds him and nurses him back to health. Why is my word not good enough?"

Still, they were adamant. I could not sway them from their official position.

I was upset and frustrated by the time I left the school. I was not sure how I was going to handle the situation; however I was sure that I was not taking Joshua to a doctor to confirm what I already knew. I tormented for hours.

My husband listened to my rage, "Why would a mother need a doctor's note? Why would a mother not have the final say in what her child is fed at school? Besides, the thought of paying Dr. Bill to write me a note to say what I already know is a waste of money. We don't have money to burn. Our money is better spent on organic food for Joshua." Ken nodded in agreement.

In my mind, there was only one reasonable answer to my questions, "A mother has the final say." Now I had to inform the school department.

I marched myself back into the principal's office with my final proposal: "I am Joshua's mom and I make the decisions what he can and cannot have in his diet. There will be no doctor's note and there will be no milk for this child either." I dared them to say otherwise. I left the office.

I am sure that was the day Joshua's file was clearly marked, "Beware of crazy mother." Truthfully, Mama Woj could turn into Mama Bear when it came to my cubs! I took great pains to keep them healthy, and no one would deny me that right.

Through this experience, Joshua became aware of just how different he was. He was the only one in his class that brought his snacks from home. His snacks were very different from what the school was serving. Instead of cookies and candy, Joshua packed trail mixes and soy yogurt (his favorite). I constantly reminded him, "Different is good. It makes you special."

Not All Corn Muffins Are Created Equal

The school was now aware that Joshua was not allowed to have milk. That was shocking enough. There was more for them to learn, and Joshua was going to teach them.

I decided it best to visit Joshua's Kindergarten teacher before school started. I wanted to be sure I had her support and hoped it would be less stressful than my meeting with the principal. I had already learned that snacks were prepared each day which consisted mostly of Kool-Aid and store-bought cookies. These foods were filled with refined sugars and hydrogenated oils, not to mention artificial colors and preservatives. Nothing on that label was good for Joshua to eat. It really was not food at all.

I explained to Joshua that this was not the kind of food that would keep him healthy. He understood. He really wasn't all that interested in cookies and Kool-Aid anyway. I don't think he even knew what Kool-Aid was. My next step was explaining it to his teacher.

"Joshua is very allergic to milk and chemicals and most of the food you serve the children contain both. It is very important that you don't feed him anything without my permission. I will make sure Joshua has a drink and snack every day from home." His teacher mostly nodded in agreement without saying much of anything.

As time went on, Joshua was coming to terms with his differences. Occasionally, he wanted to fit in, to be like everyone else. On special occasions, he would test the waters, or in this case, the food:

On the day before Thanksgiving, Joshua's teacher made a Thanksgiving feast for the class: juice and a corn muffin. Now to the naked eye, this seemed to be a very healthy snack. To Joshua, this was familiar territory. He ate corn muffins at home many times. He knew they were good for him! He was so excited that finally there was a snack

21

he could eat. What was more important, he could share the Thanksgiving feast with his classmates.

"My mom always makes corn muffins. I am sure I can have one with the class, and I always drink juice at home too!"

His teacher was leery. She heard the words in her head that I had clearly spoken. Her prime directive was, "Don't feed Joshua anything without my permission." However, I am sure that excited little face with the big bright smile was too tempting to pass up. She questioned him further.

"Yes, I am very sure it is okay. These are the things I eat at home!"

She finally consented. How bad could one corn muffin and one cup of juice be for a little guy? The decision to join in this holiday feast turned out to be the wrong one.

Joshua walked into the store that afternoon and I could tell immediately that something was drastically wrong. His face looked distorted; his eyes swollen. My first reaction was to ask, "Joshua, did you have something to eat at school today?" He was always very honest in his replies. He never had a reason to lie. He knew it was how we solved problems.

"The teacher had corn muffins and juice today, Mom. I knew those would be okay. I told her you make them all the time. So I got to have a Thanksgiving feast with my class!" He was so happy. How would I burst his little bubble?

"Honey, sit down. Mommy needs to talk to you. There is a big difference between the way Mommy cooks and teachers cook. Teachers don't know to use soy and rice milk when they make muffins. They don't know to use organic flours and whole grains, and they don't know anything about pure maple syrup and organic juices." He had no idea food was that complicated!

His face showed disappointment. There were times I wished he could be 'normal.' Except I knew in my heart, Joshua was normal. Isn't normal avoiding foods that are poisonous to sensitive little bodies? Right now, however, normal was emotionally painful.

The following day was Thanksgiving, and Joshua was in no condition to enjoy his Thanksgiving feast with his family. Unable to breathe or move, he spent the entire day on my lap.

Whether it was a combination of the milk and the chemicals that made this reaction so intense, I truly can't say. However, Joshua learned a valuable lesson. Not all corn muffins are created equal.

Reading Labels or Being Labeled?

I realize that in the real world, Joshua would have had yet another label. He would have been labeled "asthmatic." To me, he was simply allergic to milk and sensitive to chemicals which in turn caused an asthmatic reaction. He was not asthmatic; he was Joshua and Joshua was allergic to milk. Being allergic to milk can be an easy fix if you simply avoid food with milk in it. However, in the real world milk and chemicals were not so easy to avoid; they popped up everywhere.

So from time to time, he got into food that contained chemicals or dairy. From time to time, his lungs responded. I never rushed him to a hospital during one of his allergic "attacks." I kept him home and nursed him back to health.

I never thought to use a drug to help him heal. I was in fear of what a drug might do to cause more damage to his sensitive system. Instead, we learned patience. We knew through experience that these moments passed and he would improve. With each experience, Joshua grew stronger and smarter.

Joshua accepted his allergies even if the adults did not. He learned to deal with his condition by learning to say no when Mom was not around. He had to be strong because many times adults would tell him, "Just a little won't hurt." Joshua learned otherwise. Sometimes "just a little" hurt a great deal.

His teachers learned to inform me ahead of time when he needed to bring in a special snack for a special occasion. For birthday parties, Joshua had his own cakes and his own nondairy ice creams. We were learning Joshua's needs together. In the end, Joshua had to make his own choices. Each lesson taught him well.

The most important lesson I learned as a parent is that I could not heal Joshua; I could only help him heal him self. My job was to encourage him to be involved in his own healing. I could not make choices for him; I could only guide him in the right direction. To do that, I first had to be truthful with myself. I had to come to peace with the fact that even a little dairy was too much for him.

Turning to goat's milk proved to be the perfect alternative for Joshua. He did extremely well on it. He gained weight and had no reaction. Goat milk products were a much better source of calcium because they digested well and were easily absorbed into his system.

Joshua would often accompany me on our trek to the goat milk farm to buy his weekly ration. Eventually we included goat cheese and goat yogurt into his diet helping to fill his insatiable appetite. As the years went by, sheep products were added to the list of "good foods for Joshua." I searched for other healthy food sources that Joshua would eat. Some of these food sources included: sesame seeds, poppy seeds, almonds, fresh dark bitter greens and fresh green herbs.

It was effortless to sprinkle sesame seeds on Joshua's cereal or oatmeal every morning. Almond butter replaced peanut butter. Fresh herbs were easy to add to the food I cooked at dinner time, and whole grain poppy seed muffins were one of his favorite after school snacks. However, the dark bitter greens were on Joshua's "I'm not eating it" list, although many times I tried to sneak it into soups without his knowledge.

I worked endlessly to ensure Joshua's nutritional needs were met. At the same time, I loved the changes I was creating in our home. I became skilled at meal planning and enjoyed the direction our family was heading.

Chapter Three

~ Nutritional Muscle Testing ~

It would be impossible for me to write a book on healing without first citing my qualifications; or, more specifically, to explain how I was able to acquire my vast knowledge of healing techniques. Initially I was guided, or should I say commanded, into the mysterious and very misunderstood realm of kinesiology. Kinesiology is the science, though some might refer to it as more of an "art," of muscle testing.

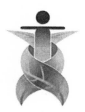

Ken and I opened our first health food store when Joshua was only six months old. This was both an exciting and a scary time for us. I had the audacity to leave my financially secure state job to become a potentially impoverished, self-sustaining proprietor. My family shook their heads in disbelief. Who could make a living on natural foods?

Ken and I felt differently. We had a mission to teach a lifestyle that had long ago been buried by chemicals and preservatives, colors and additives. We had been consciously changing our own lives over the past seven years, learning to cook food that managed to avoid alteration. We frequented nearby health food stores with bulk food departments to help make our lifestyle affordable. Containers lined our shelves filled with bulk grains, beans and dried herbs. I liked the look of our updated kitchen. I felt I had finally come home.

During this time, Ken spoke of owning his own health food store. I was willing to support his dream. Three years after moving to Connecticut the local health food store was about to close. We jumped at the opportunity to buy what was left of it and planted our feet firmly on the ground of Community Health Foods in the little village of Danielson. We were not sure if Danielson was ready for us; however, we were positive that we were ready to take on Danielson.

Our customer base was composed mostly of hippies and "druggies" and all sorts of unique individuals. This strange mix of forlorn Americana became our most trusted and committed customers. Many became our friends. The local doctors, nurses and lawyers dared not enter for fear that being recognized inside our store would place their careers in jeopardy. We often caught them staring inside our windows in awe of the strange happenings taking place inside our walls. What do people find to buy in such a strange place?

I ran the store while Ken remained at his nine to five job in the hopes of supporting all of us, including the store. Our food was different and unique. Sandwiches were made of whole grain pocket breads and goat cheese, tofu salads and sprouts. We geared our menu toward a more vegetarian fare and before long, our customer base grew. Slowly new faces ventured in; a few we saw daily. They were our first regulars. They liked what we served and we liked serving them.

David was becoming one of the regulars and on a late Tuesday afternoon he came in with an unusual request. "I am hosting a seminar at my home on muscle testing. It is being sponsored by an herb company. I think you may find it interesting, and I am sure it would benefit your business."

"What is muscle testing?" I curiously inquired.

David provided a clear and concise explanation. "Muscle testing is much like a lie detector test only it is administered through a facilitator. By applying pressure to the subject's arm, the facilitator is able to "feel" the positive or negative responses that are being communicated between the brain and the muscles. The facilitator can "read" a person by closely monitoring these responses.

A strong muscle response represents a "yes" answer and a weak muscle response represents a "no." One can ask any question that can be answered by either a yes or no response. The information sought by *the facilitator is literally at his or her fingertips, conveniently pulsing through the client."*

I politely listened to David's lengthy explanation. "It sounds fascinating; however, I don't think I am interested." Our family was already considered strange by many in the community; and this muscle testing venture could put us over the edge!

To his credit, David was not so easily deterred. About a month later, he returned. "The company is coming back to give another seminar. I know you would benefit. I think you should reconsider." I held my ground. I remained uncomfortable with the idea and again sent him away.

David is an amazing person. He seemed disinclined to accept "no" for an answer. I learned something about strength of character from him; a lesson that would serve me well in the years ahead. With a strong and confident voice, David gave it his best effort, "Linda, I really think this seminar is important. We are hosting it again. You need to be there!" Three times is a charm to many; at that moment it felt more akin to a divine offering. I decided to accept his final offer.

I finally realized that David was the messenger. It was time for me to accept the invitation. I attended the next seminar and many others that followed.

Attending David's seminar changed the direction of my life. I spoke about my experiences and people were fascinated to the point that they offered themselves as "guinea pigs" so I could practice my muscle testing techniques. I had a gift from the very beginning. Of the ten original participants in those early classes, I was the only one who continued using muscle testing to recreate myself as a Nutritional Kinesiologist and Spiritual Intuitive. The year of this life-changing experience was 1983. What I have learned since could fill a novel, but that is another story altogether.

Over the past 30 years, my practice has grown and flourished. Word of mouth is my main marketing tool. I am often approached by those who are desperately looking for the answers to their problems.

Repeatedly, I am told that I am their last hope; conventional medicine was unsuccessful in their quest to heal. I love the challenge and the opportunity to help them heal. I am quite clear however, that I cannot heal anyone. My job is to teach each client how to heal the "self."

This type of healing is not for everyone. It is for those who are ready to be responsible for their thoughts, words and actions. It is for those who are ready to heal themselves by making changes. Joshua was ready to take on that challenge. Muscle testing allowed me to help guide him through his process.

Patience Helps Healing

Learning this procedure would have a profound effect on how Joshua and I arrived at where we are today. Muscle testing allowed me to speak directly to Joshua's higher self whenever difficult issues presented themselves, including: *finding simple answers to seemingly complex problems, having a greater understanding of what was causing Joshua's strange reactions to his environment and recognizing triggers that prompted reactions.*

The brain is much like a computer, storing data that we may need in the future. Muscle testing allows me the ability to plug into that data, extracting information acquired throughout our life experiences.

By reading muscular responses, I am able to provide my clients with information that has been unconsciously stored over time. Muscle testing permitted me the opportunity to speak to Joshua's memory cells when his body was affected by chemicals. I learned to isolate ingredients that were causing him problems by asking the right questions.

Soy yogurt was one of Joshua's staple foods because it was one of the few food types that never caused a chemical reaction. We were always on the look out for new and different flavors to try. One day while Ken was placing his order through our distributor, he noticed a new flavor from Joshua's favorite soy yogurt company. He added it to our order.

Kiwi lemon arrived on the pallet and Joshua couldn't wait to try it! He quickly devoured the cup while letting me know how good this new flavor of yogurt tasted! The smile on his face quickly faded as he realized he was about to experience a chemical reaction.

Within minutes, Joshua started to feel dizzy. He had to sit to keep himself from falling. His throat began to itch, and he became fearful it might constrict. We never knew how strong or long a reaction might last; however, in this case we had a certain advantage, we knew the yogurt was the problem. The disadvantage was we didn't know why.

Joshua had eaten soy yogurt most of his life with no adverse reactions. He naturally started to worry that a key staple of his diet might have to be eliminated from his already short list of "safe foods." I thought differently, especially considering his history with this product.

"Joshua, I don't think it is the soy yogurt itself that is the issue for you. I think you may have reacted to one of the fruits used in the soy yogurt. Remember, this flavor is new to this company, and you have never reacted to any of the other flavors in the past. Their fruits are not certified organic, and I am thinking that until this point they had done a good job of using suppliers who were consciously not spraying chemicals on their fruits. Let's try muscle testing the ingredients and see if we can find one in particular that may be the problem." Joshua thought that was a good idea.

Using muscle testing, we addressed the individual ingredients on the product label. For most of the ingredient list, Joshua's response was strong and positive. However, one ingredient elicited a negative response. When I mentioned the word "lemon," Joshua's resistance weakened considerably.

My knowledge of muscle testing and my ability to administer this procedure had evolved to the point where I could safely arrive at a valid conclusion: the lemons in the yogurt were undoubtedly the problem. I could only assume they had been sprayed with a pesticide.

"I'm glad that you figured that out for me mom. I really liked that flavor. It's too bad I can't eat it any more." I wasn't so sure I agreed with his conclusion. I was thinking that this batch may not be indicative of future ones.

"We have always been able to trust this company in the past. Let's not discount this flavor so quickly. I suggest we wait a month or two and then order the same flavor again. When it comes in, I'll muscle test it on you before you eat it. Maybe the quality of lemons will improve with a new batch."

As an additional precaution, I took it upon myself to contact the company about Joshua's reaction. I was sure they would want to know, and I felt it was worth the time and effort.

Joshua learned patience. He waited the two months and then, as promised, Ken ordered the kiwi lemon soy yogurt again. Only this time, I muscle tested it before he ate it. All the ingredients tested positive. Joshua slowly ate the entire cup being conscious of possible reactions. There were none.

This was only the beginning of my journey. Throughout the years, I learned new ways to use muscle testing to help us all heal. I am forever grateful for David's persistence.

Chapter Four

~ Chemical Sensitivities ~

From the time Joshua was young, he learned how to deal with the symptoms of dairy allergies. He knew he was responsible for what he put into his body. He could avoid milk and products that contained milk with a simple procedure: read a label, omit the food. Through this practice, Joshua became disciplined. It did not take long to realize that dairy allergies would be the least of Joshua's problems.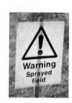

As time passed, I began to suspect that Joshua was reacting to more than just dairy. I was seeing a connection between food and his uncontrollable behaviors. Eating and drinking certain products affected his moods, and the obvious common denominator in all of these products was chemicals. I had to face the reality that my son was chemically sensitive. Identifying reactions to chemicals in his food and his environment would be our next challenge.

Chemical sensitivities proved quite different than dairy allergies. I was adept at reading labels to avoid products that contained cow dairy. I had to learn to read labels in search of chemicals hidden in our food and drink. The more I read, the more I realized that most food on the grocery shelf was not real.

Chemicals in his environment had extreme effects upon his health and could be found in unusual places. They appeared without warning and affected Joshua more harshly than anything he had experienced to date. There was much to learn about the toxic world that surrounded us. The lessons were persistent; lessons that others were incapable of grasping.

The outside world refused to understand the effects their chemicals and perfumes had on this one small child. Confusion, doubt and criticisms were becoming a way of life. Joshua had to stand strong in his beliefs especially during those times it felt uncomfortable to do so. It became more important than ever to educate those who insisted chemical sensitivities did not exist.

Tastes and smells became powerful allies. He learned to use these senses to his advantage. Through all of his experiences, Joshua became adamant about one thing: nobody knew more about Joshua than Joshua.

Abusive Behaviors

As a toddler, Joshua was a difficult child. At the dinner table, he often threw himself off of his chair and onto the floor. Many nights he did not finish his meal; he was simply sent to his room. He lashed out and struck hard when provoked. He appeared to have no control over his emotions, reacting with anger and frustration too often for my liking.

We realized this was not "normal" behavior. He had no reason to be angry and frustrated. He was not from an abusive home, and yet he constantly acted like an abused child. Consequently, our entire family felt abused by Joshua.

We tried to be patient and reason with him. We tried to get him to explain what was going on inside his head. Despite our best efforts, we sometimes got angry and frustrated, too. The only thing that calmed him was alone time in his room. Eventually, he would gain control of himself and rejoin the family; however, the new moments of calm never lasted very long and removing Joshua from the family was often the only way we found peace and solace from his abusive behaviors.

The situation was simultaneously disheartening and puzzling. Though Joshua had shown himself to be a very intelligent child, he could not be reasoned with during his rampages. During these early years, Joshua was not capable of connecting a chemical to an emotion, and I was not yet educated enough to make the connections myself.

I was at a loss to understand what was causing his severe reactions and attitude problems. However, Joshua's previous experience with dairy allergies taught me to pay close attention to him. I spent hours watching and listening as he spoke to me through his own unique language; the language of the physical and emotional bodies that we call symptoms and reactions.

I was in a constant state of awareness. When he reacted, I learned to listen to what his body was telling me. Each day brought with it a new lesson for all of us.

Most often than not, I was able to determine that Joshua's strange physical and emotional reactions could be traced back to an encounter with chemicals. It was important to find the cause of his reactions so we could deal with the problem. If we did not learn what was causing pain in the present, how could we possibly change it for the future?

I began to suspect that food might be an issue. Changes to the food we ate became a priority. As with dairy allergies, labels were our friends. If we could not read an ingredient, Joshua did not eat the product. Any label with artificial this or preservative that was immediately eliminated. His menu of acceptable foods became more limiting, yet substantially more nourishing. Joshua was discovering the meaning behind "real" food as opposed to fake food; the foods that nourished him and the foods that caused him pain. Joshua was learning to be responsible for the choices he made.

Despite all the careful precautions we both took through examination of his food and drink labels, maintaining health was still a major challenge. We had complete control over our own home and absolutely no control over anyone else's homes. He learned that chemicals were hidden in places we did not think possible. New lessons needed to be learned, and they demanded we become fast learners.

As Joshua and I discovered the multitude of chemicals that would come into his world, it became our mission to find a solution to each problem. If the cause of Joshua's chemical poisoning was connected to something in our home, we simply removed that something from our environment. If the cause was situated elsewhere within the scope of

Joshua's world, he would try to avoid the environment altogether. At times, other solutions needed to be found and not everyone was as accepting to change as we were. Our goal was always the same, however. Whatever it took to ensure Joshua's health and safety was our first priority.

The New Rug

We purchased our first health food store when Joshua was six months old. If I was working, Joshua was working with me. The front window soon turned into a playroom filled with toys and snacks that made Joshua feel at home.

By the time he was three years old, the hard wooden floor at the store had aged miserably over time and was in need of serious upgrading. However, since we did not own the building, Ken and I did not particularly want to invest too much money on the needed repairs. We opted for the quick and inexpensive solution. We had a new rug installed to cover the floor below. It did not take long to learn that the easy and cheap solutions may not always be the best when Joshua is concerned.

The day after the rug was installed Joshua was back at work with me. His eyes grew big as he recognized that there was something new at the store. It took him no time at all to feel the softness of the rug beneath his small knees. It was a huge upgrade from the hard wooden floor he was used to. He spent the first few hours of the morning crawling and rolling all over the new carpet. His joy filled the store. I was certain we made the right choice.

Then out of nowhere, Joshua was crying uncontrollably. I ran to him, "What happened?" I asked. "Did you hurt yourself?"

"No, I did not hurt myself; I don't know why I am crying," a strange reply for a three year old. He cried for a long time. It seemed as though it went on for hours, tears rolling down his face, big sad sobs, and no explanation. He could see I was looking to him for answers. His

only reply was, *"I can't help it. I can't stop."* Joshua was being truthful; he had lost control of himself.

Customers came and went, each asking, *"What is wrong with Josh?"*

"We are not sure," was the only answer I could give them. Joshua continued to cry and I couldn't help but wonder what our customers were thinking.

Then another thought entered my mind. The new rug! As with any *"new"* introduction into Joshua's space, a reaction always indicated that a chemical had invaded his environment. I quickly realized the rug was the culprit. It was the only new item he had encountered that day. I had not given any thought to the fact that new rugs contain formaldehyde. I was embarrassed to admit that I poisoned my own son.

As I held Joshua and tried to console him, I had another thought. Were tears a way of helping him discharge the chemical from his body? Perhaps this was not a pleasant way, but it was effective nonetheless. So I encouraged him to let it all out, as much as he could to avoid the possibility of more intense symptoms later.

As I helped Joshua through his stream of tears, my next thought was, *"How do I fix the problem I have created?"*

I was learning that Joshua was my little computer. His reactions were signals letting me know we had a problem. If the chemicals in the rug had this profound effect upon him, could they also be affecting me and every customer who entered the store? Joshua's reaction was undeniable. Were others not so noticeable? Joshua was there to inform me, and I began to reason that if a chemical affected Joshua, it affected everyone.

I needed to solve this problem. I loved having Joshua with me at the store. He was my coworker and partner. We worked, or should I say played, great together. What was more important, I was his mother. I could not continue to poison him. I was not going to let a rug interfere with the time we spent together.

My first thought was to get rid of anything that caused Joshua a problem. Eliminate the rug from his environment. That would certainly solve the problem, and without much hassle. Yet the rug was important to the look and feel of the store. We bought the rug because we needed it. The very idea of undoing what we had just done did not seem quite right to me, and the cost played an ever so slight role. It was not like we had extra money sitting in our account for Plan B. I searched my mind for another solution. I am a great believer in, "Ask and you shall receive."

The solution soon came to me as an old recipe; only this recipe was not for cooking, it was for washing. It was as though someone spoke to me inside my head and I heard clearly: "lemon juice and baking soda."

At this point I thought, "What do I have to lose? Either it will work or it won't." I wasn't sure if lemon juice and baking soda could fix the chemical problem; however, I knew it was better than doing nothing, so Plan C was set into action.

To this day, I can't tell you how I knew about that recipe. I might have read it somewhere or heard it in passing. I prefer to think, however, that the angels were listening and wanted to help a three year old boy who needed healing. Regardless of how I acquired that essential bit of information, I did not wait to act upon it.

I took Joshua home and headed to the nearest market to rent a carpet cleaner minus the chemical detergents. I knew that would not help our situation in the least bit.

At the rental counter, the person behind the desk was insistent, "You need to buy the cleaning solutions for the carpet cleaner to work." I was sure I needed something else. I left the store with the machine, a box of baking soda and a bottle of lemon juice.

My next dilemma was, "How much do I use of each?" I had nothing but my intuition to go on. It was not like we could Google back then. I winged it! Half a cup of this; half a cup of that making sure the water was hot enough to dissolve the baking soda. Then I began to thoroughly wash our new carpet with my natural cleaning solution.

It was late by the time I left the store. I breathed in a scent of clean lemon smell. I hoped it worked as I shut off the lights to go home.

Back at home, I found Joshua upstairs in his room. He was getting ready for bed and seemed to have no more noticeable reaction. "I cleaned the carpet at the store tonight," I informed him. "Would you like to try to come to work with me in the morning?"

I could tell by the look on his face he was not sure if that was a good idea. As young as he was, he did have an opinion about his health. "I don't want to go if the rug is going to make me cry some more. I did not like that."

"I know and if you feel it is affecting you, I promise to take you right home. How will we know unless we try?" I was putting all my faith into my lemon juice and baking soda formula. If it did not work, the rug would have to go. Joshua's health was definitely more important.

Joshua returned to the store with me the next day. He was very cautious and avoided getting too close to the rug. He stood by my side for a long time while we waited for any reaction. I naturally paid close attention to him; he was doing the same. After a long while, we both became more comfortable that there would be no tears or emotional outbursts. Ever so slowly he made his way to the front window and by the end of the day he was back laughing and playing on his new carpet.

We learned a valuable lesson that day. If we search, and ask, we may find a solution to the problem presented. Joshua may not be able to live comfortably in the "real" world of chemicals and poisons; however, by taking different steps, he can continue to live healthy in our world. I now knew that I could indeed buy new rugs for our home and for our store; I just had to wash away the chemicals before Joshua could play on them.

Joshua's tears were only one symptom of chemical poisoning. As time went on, we would learn that Joshua experienced many symptoms, both physical and emotional.

Out Go the Cleaning Products

The experience with the rug was a huge reality check. It opened up new questions and concerns. If a chemical in the rug affected Joshua so severely, were equal or greater quantities of chemicals in our home also affecting him at some level? Do all chemicals affect him no matter how minute? Could the chemicals I use for cleaning, polishing and washing be part of the problem that influenced his abusive behaviors? My instincts told me it was worth investigating.

I spent the rest of that week going through cupboards and drawers. I checked all my cleaning products, polishes, hair sprays; you name it. If it looked, smelled or acted like a chemical, it was promptly replaced with a natural alternative. I was on a mission to clean up our environment for the good of all of us, especially Joshua.

Joshua watched as the garbage can was filled and the cupboards were emptied. I took this time to share my thoughts and feelings with him. "If a rug can cause you to have an emotional response, Mom is thinking that the chemicals we use everyday may be doing the same, except in a different way. Suppose some of these products we spray around our home are adding to your behavior problems. What if these products are harmful to all of us? The only way we will know for sure is if we try something new, and that is what Mom is doing."

I subsequently educated myself about natural ingredients. Products such as Murphy's Oil Soap and Arm and Hammer laundry detergent began to fill my cupboards. Instead of getting upset about having to alter our lives, I used that energy to make the changes I deemed necessary. I ordered more natural cleaning products at the store and soon our home was feeling and smelling chemical free.

As I think back, it never occurred to me to store these products in case my theory was incorrect. At some level, I was certain these chemicals were playing havoc with Joshua's system, and I knew they were not coming back into my home. They were leaving for good and I was making sure of it.

In no time, I witness a marked improvement in Joshua's behavior. He was spending less time in his room and more time with us at the dinner table. The energy of our home was becoming more balanced and happy. Joshua was starting to feel safe and secure. So was the rest of our family.

This was a life altering day. We understood the changes we would have to commit to as a family to ensure Joshua's happy state of mind and we were willing to go the extra yards. Joshua would be fully supported by all of us.

Don't Drink The Water!

The water Joshua drinks cannot be tainted with rust inhibitors, chlorine or fluoride. It must be pure. Drinking water that is contaminated with chemicals can have profound negative effects, especially to a chemically sensitive child like Joshua.

One of Joshua's earliest symptoms of chemical poisoning was anger and rage. As Joshua learned to recognize the chemicals that triggered these emotions, we were able to avoid them by replacing chemicals in our home with natural alternatives. With each change, the frequency and volume of his outbursts dissipated.

Changes to his food and environment were essential, and the introduction of alternative medicines helped to further improve his behavior. He was happier and healthier for all our efforts. Every so often, however, his nasty behavior resurfaced. We used these opportunities to learn more about how his body reacted to certain outside influences.

Joshua was seven years old. It was September of his second year of elementary school. Shortly after school began, Joshua's behavior became violent. He came home every day and would literally start banging his head on the floor boards. I could not reason with him, nor could he explain what might be causing these violent outbursts. I had not seen this behavior since we cleaned up our environment and our food years ago.

Each day I bombarded him with the same basic series of questions. "Do you smell anything strange at school? Is anyone painting in or around the school? Did they install new rugs on the floors?" We were all too familiar with the common triggers that often caused these behaviors.

His acute sense of smell had always helped in solving these dilemmas. This time, even Joshua was baffled. "No, Mom. There's nothing that smells strange at school. I don't know why I am acting this way. I can't control myself." He was right. He had no control over himself. He was angry and the pain he felt within was being played out through his actions. Spending alone time in his room was the only way he was able to calm down and gain control of him self.

As the behavior continued into the next week, my questions took on a greater urgency. I started delving into alternative areas of possible explanation. "Is anyone using something different in class? Does the teacher spray anything in the classroom? Can you smell any fumes or chemicals?" All I received in response were the same answers. He did not recognize anything that was unfamiliar or strange in his environment. Each afternoon, he was back in his room. How long could this go on?

By dinner time, Joshua's behavior shifted, and weekends were free of rage. That confirmed my suspicions that something at school was the trigger. I did not like the idea of him spending entire afternoons alone in his room, yet I could not stand to watch him abuse himself. Similarly, I did not wish to be abused by him either.

After many weeks of the entire family having to endure this roller-coaster ride, Joshua made a single statement that helped to solve his problem. "Mom, the water at school tastes funny."

The water tastes funny? Could that be the problem? Could he really "taste" something strange in the water? I began to reason that if his sense of smell was acute, why would his sense of taste be any different? A feeling of hope overcame me.

I was elated and quickly replied, "Stop drinking the water!" We sat and talked about the importance of this single statement. "Your sense of smell has always helped you recognize chemicals that affect you. Now your sense of taste is letting you know that you have another ally to help you heal. This is exciting. I am so happy you finally shared this information with me. Now what do we do about it?"

From the look on his face, Joshua was confused. Yes, the water tasted strange for awhile; however, he had no choice but to drink the water the school supplied. A trip to the bubbler was a ceremonial experience each day and the class participated together.

"Mom, I have to drink the water. I can't go all day without water." Joshua was a big water drinker. Water helped him flush chemicals and toxins through his system. However, if water were the problem, was it really helping him?

"You're right Josh. You do have to drink water. However, you cannot drink water that may be making you ill. Tomorrow I will fill a bottle with our water and you can drink that instead."

That was way too weird for Joshua. He already had to take all his own snacks and lunch into school. Everyone else shared the same snack; his was always different. Everyone else bought lunch; he always carried a lunch box. Now a water bottle too?

"If we don't do this, how will you know? How will you get better? Would you rather continue throwing yourself on the floor?"

That did not sit well with Joshua. He did not like spending every afternoon in his room. He was ready to heal.

"Okay, Mom. I need to know too."

The next day, Joshua left home armed with two items: a bottle with water from our well and a note for his teacher.

"Dear Ms. ____. I think Joshua is experiencing a reaction from the water at school. Please allow him to bring in his own water for a few weeks to see if it helps improve his behavior."

At that time, bringing water to school was not deemed an acceptable practice. The city water supplies were considered safe. Conversely, Joshua was considered strange and malady susceptible.

It no longer mattered to me what others might think. All that mattered was finding a solution to the problem that Joshua was experiencing. My son needed safe drinking water during the day and the school system was not supplying it. The solution was obvious; supply our own. Joshua understood that the bubbler was no longer an option, so he always kept a bottle of water with him and opted out of the daily bubbler ritual. Joshua was opting out before it was fashionable.

Joshua's attitude changed overnight. He was suddenly coming home from school happy and sharing his day at the dinner table. His temper tantrums disappeared. He was proud of himself for having identified the problem. He no longer cared that others might think him weird. Pure water was important to his health and he trusted his water at home. Eventually, it was the only water he was willing to drink.

This was a transcendental moment. Joshua was now able to clearly see that being special was a gift and not a curse. His gift allowed him to learn more about himself and what was causing him to misbehave. It was another example of how the power of healing originates within.

Joshua did not want to be angry. He preferred happiness and contentment. Once he recognized the cause of his problem, he felt empowered to fix it. From that day on, Joshua knew enough to pay attention to both his sense of taste and his sense of smell. For my part, I felt the need to explain to his teacher what was happening with Joshua and the water at school.

The following week, I called the school to make an appointment to meet with Joshua's teacher. I knew that our family was considered very strange, and bringing water to school was a strange request. I brought her up to date. As my story unfolded about the correlation between Joshua's behavior and the bubbler, she could not help but smile.

"There is no need to explain. Since Joshua has been bringing in his own water to school, I too have seen a marked improvement in his behavior. Not only that, since he stopped drinking from the bubbler, his grades have gone up!"

That was an important confirmation for Joshua. He knew his behavior had improved, but did not realize that his performance in school had improved as well. That single statement from his teacher opened Joshua's eyes to many new possibilities. Most significantly, he started paying attention to how certain chemicals might affect his ability to learn and to focus.

It also made Joshua feel good to have the support of his teacher. Henceforth, he no longer felt weird about bringing water from home to drink in school. From this one episode, I could not help but wonder, "How many other children were being affected in the same way?" I did not believe that Joshua was unique to this situation.

Joshua possessed a unique ability to "listen" through his senses. This is an ability that many of us once possessed, but which the vast majority have clearly lost or forgotten. The story did not end there:

Later that year, our local water company sent out a special notice to all of its customers. This notice was placed in the same envelope that contained the company's quarterly water bills. The notice politely informed customers that there had been a chemical spill in one of their wells. It went on to say that there was no real need for concern, because the problem had already been solved. It seems the solution to this problem was simply to increase the safety standards for that particular chemical.

Pure water is fast becoming a commodity of the past and the lack of pure water is indeed a huge problem. The solution to this problem was to convince everyone that drinking chemicals is acceptable.

Joshua was being greatly affected by drinking water that was poisoning his system. A chemical spill in a water supply is a nightmare; changing standards to accommodate this nightmare is akin to a horror movie.

I spoke vehemently about this situation, but few seemed to care. Though I could not force change on the many, I could initiate change within myself. I could also teach my children what I knew to be true. Pure water is essential to a healthy mind and body. Today, my entire family is conscious about the water we drink and avoid any water that may be purified or contaminated with chemicals.

Symptoms of Chemical Poisoning

Chemical reactions come in many shapes and sizes. Joshua probably experienced all of them at one time or another throughout his healing.

Some common symptoms of Joshua's chemical sensitivities even to this day are: *Skin rashes, asthma, swollen glands, cysts, boils, inability to concentrate, irrational behavior, sinusitis, headaches, hives, exhaustion, and dizziness.*

The intensity of the reaction was often connected to the type of chemical and the length of the exposure. Sometimes Joshua would be able to tell immediately how bad the reaction was from the initial moment he was exposed. His body was like a temperature gauge, rising quickly to changes in his food, water and environment.

Many of the symptoms Joshua experienced are the same ones many children today are experiencing. If we were to recognize these symptoms as chemical poisoning, our lives will be greatly altered and chemical medicines could never be the cure; they would become part of the problem.

Joshua entered the world with a pure body, heart and mind. It did not take long to poison all three by unconsciously feeding him tainted food and water as well as introducing him into an environment surrounded with chemicals and poisons. To help him heal, I learned to make choices that ensured him pure food, clean water and a safe environment.

Chemical Free Zones or Is It Homes?

I firmly believe that if Joshua lived with a typical American family, he would have been labeled ADHD from the moment he entered a classroom. When poisoned by chemicals, he had all the classic symptoms ascribed to ADHD children: Irrational behaviors, inability to concentrate, lack of focus. Joshua was a sure candidate for that label.

Yet, the only label I would allow anyone to give him was "chemically sensitive." For all of his behavior imbalances, chemical poisoning was commonly the culprit.

Luckily, we were not a typical American family. I did not run to doctors for help unless it was Joshua's homeopathic physician. I refused to use drugs as a means to control him. Instead I wanted to learn from him. I wanted him to be able to express to me what the real issues were that caused such behaviors and attitudes.

As a family, we chose to opt out of the "drug" plan and into the "chemical-free" plan. We chose to eliminate poisons and chemicals from our home. It was a decision that was a blessing.

Avoiding chemicals in our own home was easy; avoiding them in other's homes was not so easy. Joshua had to be careful about the world he walked through. Around many twists and turns, a chemical was waiting to enter his space. Trying to educate people that chemicals were detrimental to Joshua's health was a difficult task. Like dairy products, friends and family were accustomed to their chemicals and could not understand how one substance could affect a young boy so harshly.

Our family may have been different from most, but we were not naive. We understood that people were more comfortable with the label of ADHD than they were with chemical sensitivities. We learned to honor their beliefs. Our beliefs were extremely different. Family and friends watched as our entire lifestyle needing altering. They had no desire or intention of following our leads. It did not deter me, however, from trying to educate them about what Joshua was teaching me.

I tried to influence those closest to us. Joshua spent a great deal of time with our friends and families, and he needed their support as well as ours. I did not expect them to change for him; I did expect them to honor the truth about his sensitivities. If they chose chemicals over Joshua's needs I asked to be told about this beforehand so Joshua could avoid a possible impending illness. There were some homes we simply expected to be safe, and that was a big mistake.

One beautiful spring day, we took a ride to my Mom and Dad's home for a short visit. There was a large blue ball sitting out on their front lawn, an unexpected surprise. Joshua scrambled to get out of the car.

"Grammy has a ball on the lawn. Can I play with it?" I was sure it was intended for the children and he was soon outside bouncing the ball around Grammy's small driveway and running through the front lawn. Joshua never needed the attention of others to enjoy life. He was content playing by himself. I watched from the window. He was having such a good time that we stayed much later than anticipated.

When it was time to leave, we pulled out of my parents' driveway. It was at that moment that a small sign on the front lawn caught my attention. I stretched to read its words. Something about that sign was familiar and I could feel pangs of nervousness throughout my body.

"Ken, please turn the car around so I can read that sign." As he started to comply, my gut was already reciting its message into my ears, "Pesticide Application."

I was shocked! My mother was aware of Joshua's sensitivities. We had numerous conversations about his reactions to chemicals in his environment. I was not upset that my mother chose to spray her lawn. That was understandably her choice to make. The problem was that she failed to disclose this information and allowed Joshua to play on grass covered with poisons.

What people do in their own homes or to their own lawns would normally not affect Joshua. However, this particular application was sure to affect him. He was literally rolling in it. Had we been notified in advance, we could have chosen not to visit my parents. Worst case, I could have kept Joshua from playing on the lawn. My frustration resulted from not being presented with the option to choose what was best for my son.

By evening, Joshua was beginning to experience the symptoms of chemical poisoning, and by bedtime, he was very ill. His glands were swollen, making it difficult for him to breathe. His constitutional remedy normally would help to lessen the severity of the symptoms quickly; however, this was not the case this time. His symptoms lasted for five long days. We both knew we could do nothing but wait. Joshua and I waited together.

It was a scenario we often played out during these situations. An inability to breathe created fear, and he did not want to be left alone. Together we would sit on a couch or he would sit on my lap. I was the support system he knew he could count on.

By the third day, his symptoms shifted. As always, we knew he would get better. His body was strong and determined, and his homeopathic remedies and cleansing herbs helped to slowly work the chemical through his system. Eventually, his symptoms lessened, and by the sixth day, they finally disappeared altogether.

I was angry. This was an illness that could have been avoided! I called my mother and explained the situation. "Mom, why didn't you tell me that you sprayed your lawn? Joshua is sick from playing on those pesticides. He can't breathe; his throat is constricted. He is afraid to go to your house."

My poor mother could not apologize enough. She knew it was not the right thing to do and yet she chose to hide her choice from us. "It is your yard, Mom. I don't want to tell you what to do on your property; however, if you choose to spray chemicals Joshua can't come over. It is too painful an experience and it's just not worth it to him."

In retrospect, I know she wished she told us about the application. She was upset that her lack of communication caused Joshua physical pain. That was something she never meant to happen. Like dairy products, Joshua's grandmother did not believe chemicals could have such a profound effect on a person.

She called back the following day, "I cancelled my contract with the lawn company. Joshua does not have to be afraid to come and play any more."

Joshua was elated with the fact that his grandmother was honoring him for who he was. Joshua could now feel secure at his grandparents' home. I was grateful that my mother decided to put Joshua's health above the appearance of her lawn.

I realize that healthy lawns are an important aspect of many people's lives, and decisions are often made to apply chemicals to them. I believe the health of a child should take precedence.

The warning signs regarding the presence of such dangerous chemicals are so small that they often go unnoticed. This was certainly the case when we first arrived at my mom's house, even though we are conscious observers. The ball obviously had our full attention. Trivial signs to announce a chemical application should not equate to trivial thoughts about the chemicals being applied.

Kill Those Bugs!

By the time Joshua was seven years old, he was venturing further away from the safety of our home. He liked his new found freedom. He was feeling confident and maintained his health by making healthy choices. One day he was invited to spend the day at a campground with family and friends. He was leaving home without me.

Joshua was excited. We packed food and drinks in a backpack and he waited for my cousin to pick him up for a day of campfires, swimming and hiking. Joshua loved the great out of doors. He couldn't wait for the day to begin.

I was excited for him that his life was becoming more "normal." What trouble could he get into with nature? That was where he always felt safe and secure. The plants and animals had no negative effects on him, and the campground they were going to was deep in the rural woods of Connecticut. A safe haven for everyone!

As daylight turned to dusk, Joshua returned home. He entered the back door full of stories about the woods and the streams, swimming and hiking. He obviously had a wonderful time.

Shortly after arriving home, however, he knew something was wrong. His entire body broke out in a severe rash. It quickly appeared everywhere, on his hands, arms, belly, back and legs. It looked serious.

I began the list of usual questions under these circumstances: "Did you eat anything at the campground? Did you drink anything that wasn't in your backpack? Did you notice any unusual smells?" Joshua just shook his head. Nothing came to mind. He had no answers for me.

I decided to call my cousin who attended to Joshua's needs that day. I wanted to find out exactly what was causing his reaction. Something was amiss here, and it helped me to know what Joshua was dealing with. "Could there have been chemicals around the campground?" I asked.

She cautiously answered, "Well, we did spray insect repellent all around the area because we were being bothered by mosquitoes." From what I gathered they had fumigated the entire area, a fog of chemicals surrounding everyone. I was surprised that Joshua had not gotten a whiff of the chemical scent. Maybe he was not there during the initial spraying or maybe he was having too much fun to notice, and maybe that was best. It did not upset his day and what would a young child do at that point but worry about what was to come? It was best he was unaware. The appearance of Joshua's body rash was now making sense to me.

The rash was severe enough to warrant a call to Joshua's homeopathic physician. I wanted to make sure I did everything necessary before the possibility the reaction might interfere with his breathing in any way.

I explained the situation at the campground to Dr. Bill and described Joshua's reaction from the exposure to the chemical. It was important to keep Dr. Bill informed. A log of reactions to various stimuli might prove helpful in the future.

I already gave Joshua a dose of his constitutional remedy. It was always the first thing I did when symptoms from chemicals appeared. I was hoping I could give him more if need be. Dr. Bill agreed that an extra dose might prove beneficial. Within hours of receiving the second dose, the rash began to diminish; by morning it was completely gone.

Joshua turned out to be a human casualty in a much larger war that seemingly goes on without an end in sight: the ongoing war against bugs. I was fortunate to have the correct antidote handy to help my son heal faster. I shudder when I watch a parent spray chemical bug repellents on a child. That one act could have devastating effects on Joshua.

Without homeopathy, I often wondered if I would have been tempted to take Joshua to a hospital to alleviate some of his maladies. At times, his symptoms were certainly severe enough; however, I knew there was nothing an allopathic doctor could do except to prescribe a chemical drug. That was unacceptable. The allopathic doctor's idea of a cure could be worse than the symptom.

Perfumes Are Chemicals Too!

Headaches are another symptom of chemical sensitivities. For Joshua they were often connected to strong smelling scents and odors. Anything that emitted a chemical smell created an instant headache. Dizziness and inability to concentrate often accompanied the headache. It was a challenge for Joshua to avoid these scents; and because chemically sensitive individuals have an acute sense of smell, he usually whiffed it in the air long before anyone else could.

Due to his extreme reactions, I once considered hanging a sign on my door that read, "If you're wearing perfumes, you can't come in." I never did, of course, because how weird could we get? Yet watching Joshua suffer in his own home was a lot to bear.

Our family and friends eventually learned to keep their cosmetics at home when visiting. I'm sure we insulted everyone at least once. However, those who truly loved Joshua respected our nontoxic space without complaint.

I am a firm believer in the saying, "What we avoid, we will attract." So it did not surprise me when perfumes came knocking at our door:

My best friend, Kathy, was between homes and needed a place to stay for a few months. Kathy had always been respectful of our lifestyle and our home had plenty of room to accommodate her. We happily obliged her request.

New people bring with them new friends. One day, Kathy's friend, Janice, stopped by for a visit. I am not gifted with the best sense of smell; however, a strong and mostly unpleasant perfume odor greeted me at the door. My mind said, "Oh no!" and my mouth said, "Come in." What else could I do? I did not even know this person and she certainly had no prior knowledge of our weirdness. Get ready for weirdo lesson #1.

Janice smelled as though she was covered from head to toe with all sorts of cosmetic sprays, none of them natural, all of them chemical. The scents followed her around like a skunk in fear. Wherever she walked, the scents lingered behind. "Yuck" was all I could think. Was Janice aware of the smells she emitted?

Janice was creating a huge problem for Joshua. Within minutes of her arrival Joshua's head began to ache, and he became nauseous and dizzy. There was a look of horror on his face; I stood dumbfounded, wondering how to approach this sensitive subject without completely embarrassing Janice and my friend.

As the moments passed without a word from me, Joshua made a quick exit and ran up to his room. He dared not come down and stayed upstairs for the evening, undoubtedly fearful of prolonging his symptoms. Janice and her smells lurked on the lower level long after she was gone.

Joshua essentially had become a prisoner in his own home. This wasn't acceptable. Of any place he ventured, he should always feel safe at home.

My friend Kathy was quite aware of what was happening. She just wasn't sure what to do either. I decided to approach Janice as gently as I could. "I'm not sure how to say this, Janice, so I guess I need to get right to the point." Janice stared at me, unsure of who I was and what I might have to say. "My son is extremely sensitive, and the perfumes you wear are making him ill. He can't be near you without getting a headache."

Janice stood there with her mouth on the floor. She had no idea how to respond to me. I just told her she smelled! She waited knowing there was more to come. "I need your help. The next time you visit, would you mind avoiding the perfumes and cosmetics with heavy smells?" I had to wonder, would there even be a next time? In her mind I am sure she thought us all crazy, and who would Janice be without her vast array of scents? I smiled just thinking about it.

Janice gave me a strange look, but assured me that she understood the problem. I was grateful that our conversation went so smoothly. She stayed for a little while and visited with Kathy. After she left, it took some time before her scents began to dissipate. Joshua refused to show his face on the first floor until the next morning. Much like a war zone, he had to be sure the enemy was long gone. The enemy was not Janice; the enemy was perfume

Janice made a great effort to adhere to our request. With each visit, however, one thing became obvious. Even without her daily spraying ritual, the odor of perfume lingered on her body and clothing. Janice could not get rid of her smells. What more could I do? Try as she might, she could not truly rid herself of that odor. Consequently, Joshua could not possibly rid himself of the reactions he suffered whenever she was around. I wonder if Janice noticed that Joshua disappeared with each visit.

Fumes were also detrimental to Joshua's health. On a normal drive, we challenged ourselves to avoid getting behind a diesel truck, which would force him to inhale the remnants of all kinds of noxious gases. A diesel truck could cost Joshua a headache for the duration of our trip.

Out Goes The Kitty Litter!

According to The National Center for Biotechnology Information website, "Hives are raised, often itchy, red welts on the surface of the skin. They are usually an allergic reaction to food or medicine." Someone forgot to tell them that hives are also triggered by poisons entering the body through the environment.

By the time Joshua entered middle school, his body was reacting in different ways to different chemicals. The fastest way to discharge a chemical is through the skin. The skin is used as a filter when the liver and spleen are overburdened, and Joshua's liver and spleen were often in an overburdened state of toxicity.

His skin was quick to react when a new chemical entered his environment. Because chemicals come in so many forms, every so often one would slip into our home unconsciously. We admittedly made plenty of mistakes, and Joshua's body made sure we took steps to immediately remedy the situation.

Winter arrived with a vengeance the year Joshua turned twelve. It was cold outside. Holly Beth was worried about her cat. "Mom, it is way too cold. Gracie could freeze out there! Why can't we get a litter box?"

I never fancied litter boxes. I did not like the mess and I especially did not like the odors. Holly Beth assured me, "I promise I will take care of it." How many times had I heard those words? Yet, she was right. It was way too cold for Gracie to be in that extreme weather. It was way too cold for anyone to be outside. I relented, reminding her of her promise.

Holly Beth and I went to the store later that day. She was happy to get her wish. She loved all her animals intensely. We quickly picked out a name brand of kitty litter that we recognized as well as a plastic litter box and liners. Holly Beth took care of setting it up and showing Gracie exactly what was expected of her.

Gracie seemed content with her new arrangement and quickly learned how to use the box. A few days later, she padded her way into Joshua's room. This was unusual behavior in itself, because Gracie was not particularly friendly toward Joshua and they rarely gave attention to one another.

Joshua was busy getting ready for school and paid little attention to the cat. He was standing in his bare feet searching for socks. The cat was being very affectionate, brushing up against Joshua's feet and legs looking for his attention. Very strange! Within a matter of moments, Joshua's feet were covered with hives. He charged into my room scratching both feet and screaming. "Mom, my feet are all broken out. I can't stop itching!" He was quick to remember that the cat had just brushed up against that very spot.

"That's strange," I said. "The cat never bothered you before."

"What about the cat litter?" he asked.

I realized that I had not read the product label before making our purchase. It never occurred to me that cat litter could be so toxic. What was I thinking? I immediately checked the label. Sure enough, the cat litter was loaded with chemicals to avoid smells and bacteria. The chemicals from the cat litter ended up on the cat's feet, and then were transferred onto Joshua's feet through Gracie's need for attention. "Wash off your feet. I'll take care of the litter box." Out went the kitty litter, and Joshua's hives soon disappeared.

Later that day, Holly Beth and I were back at the store reading kitty litter labels. We found one that we felt would solve our problem. Gracie and Joshua personally tested it for its affects. No hives; no problem! I *can only assume that Gracie was happier and healthier because of our choice as well.*

Joshua became our barometer for determining what was healthy and what was not. We learned through his reactions. Although it was clearly not easy for Joshua to experience all kinds of symptoms, we were all learning about the importance of a clean environment. As we changed for him, we were also changing for ourselves. Having a cleaner home was a gift bestowed upon the entire family.

Chapter Five

~ A Heaping of Health Food ~

The health food industry that existed in the mid-1980s was far from mainstream, but Ken and I were passionate about getting involved. Our store connected me to food choices that were considered "strange" at the time. Whole grains, fresh organic fruits and vegetables, nuts, seeds and beans had lost favor with most families. These foods were considered too time-consuming for a public that was readily buying into the new-age mentality of "faster is better." Eating out, rather than eating in, afforded many families a new social experience.

Our new social experience was our store and customers quickly became family and friends. The store was taking on an identity of its own and before long it became a school for alternative eating and living. As the store grew, so did our knowledge of food and its varied affects on the body and mind. Each day was a new learning experience, which I was always happy to share with anyone who showed a remote interest.

I felt it was not by chance that we were led into the health food industry. The store allowed us to buy quality food at reasonable prices. Joshua's insatiable appetite could have set us in the poor house, even poorer than we were at the time.

Because we chose to dramatically change our lives, we were no longer enamored with the luxury of eating out. Money was tight; eating at home was affordable. I learned to cook slow food before the slow food movement became a fad. Even better, I discovered I enjoyed this new way of preparing food for my family. As we continued to learn more about Joshua's sensitivities, home cooking was often our only option.

Joshua's sensitivities mandated knowing what was in the food. Anything unnatural was capable of triggering a reaction. The only way to ensure we were eating pure food was to make it myself with ingredients I knew to be pure. The more I understood about the importance of quality food, the more I wanted to cook at home.

Through trial and error, I learned how to steam and roast fresh organic vegetables. I learned how to cook whole grains and beans. Nuts and seeds became a staple, and organic fresh fruit was the main ingredient in my cakes, cookies and pies. My cupboards were free of artificial colors, flavorings and sweeteners, as well as refined sugars, flours and hydrogenated oils. I was choosing what went into my children's mouths and the choices I made felt good. Yes, this all took a great deal of my time and energy; however, I found this to be a wonderful and valuable way to be spending both!

Joshua was sensitive to so many ingredients that I became uncomfortable when other people wanted to cook for him. Eating away from home often resulted in some type of reaction. It just wasn't worth the trouble. When I cooked at home, Joshua felt safe. He knew what was in the food, and he knew it would not have an adverse effect. Feeling safe kept him balanced and helped him heal.

If we were the type of family that opted for fast food over home cooking, Joshua would not have had the opportunity to discover so much about his sensitive nature. Worse, he would have remained in a relatively constant state of sickness. The better the quality of the food Joshua ate and the cleaner we kept his environment, the healthier he became, physically, emotionally and mentally.

This is not to say we never dined out. However, when we did, deciding where we ate was important. Food was a major investment in Joshua's health, so the restaurants we frequented had to be as conscious about using pure ingredients as we were. There were a handful of local restaurants Joshua enjoyed, but his unequivocal favorite place to eat was in our own kitchen.

Strawberries Sweet and Toxic

Traveling could be challenging. When on the road, we searched for health food stores that included cafes or small family owned restaurants with healthy menus. If we made a bad choice, we knew it soon enough. Chemicals come in many shapes and sizes, and Joshua's body always clued us in to where they were hidden. The story of how a fresh bowl of strawberries turned detrimental opened my eyes to just how toxic our food can be:

When Joshua was five years old, we took a weekend trip to New Hampshire. On our way home, everyone was getting hungry, so we searched for an acceptable place to eat. My idea of an "acceptable" restaurant was not always in line with the rest of the family. We avoided fast food places. The children had given up asking. So it was not always easy to agree on what would meet all our needs and taste buds.

We learned through experience that some of the little villages along the way may offer options that were suitable. We eventually found a small health food restaurant. It was our routine to check out menus before committing to eating anywhere.

After scouring the menu, Ken and I were happy with the selections; the children were not, especially Joshua. "Why do we have to eat here? "There's nothing good on the menu." However, I felt it had all the earmarks of a safe choice for Joshua and his sensitivities.

Joshua was used to limitations when it came to food. Menus could be even more limiting, which I understood was frustrating for him. I began reading off selections that I thought might interest him. He became very disagreeable. After way too many, "No, I don't want that" answers, my final offer was a bowl of fresh strawberries. Joshua's eyes lit up. "I'll have that!"

The strawberries arrived plump and juicy. Joshua was happy which helped make the rest of us happy as well. We finished lunch and headed out to the car. By the time Joshua was at the car door, his eyes were filled with tears. "What happened?" I asked.

Shannon looked at me with confusion. "I didn't do anything," she assured me.

It did not take long to realize something was drastically wrong. His tears were starting to stream down his face with uncontrollable sobs. "Josh, why are you crying?"

"I don't know," he replied. "I can't help myself."

These are words I heard before. Joshua could not help himself. He had absolutely no control over this outpouring of emotions. I tried to reason with him even though I knew it would not help the situation. Whatever was affecting him would channel through his body in its own time. All I could do was comfort him through the experience.

The crying lasted for almost an hour. While I waited I wondered how to tell him I thought he might be allergic to strawberries. His choices were limited as it was, and I would have to delete another food from his diminishing list of "foods that were safe for Joshua to eat." Eventually he calmed himself down and we continued our ride home without incident.

A month or so later, the strawberry patch that I planted the year before was now bursting with ripe, red berries. From my kitchen window, I spotted Joshua in the middle of the patch feasting on the tasty fruits. Along side the strawberries were snap peas filled with green pods. I watched as he alternated strawberries and pea pods for an afternoon snack. How quickly he forgot his emotional trauma from the month before. Such is the joy of childhood.

I resigned myself to the fact that he and I would be in for an emotional afternoon. To my surprise, however, Joshua suffered no reaction at all. Just the opposite occurred. He was in a great mood, happy and content. His belly was full!

That's when I realized it was not the strawberries that caused his reaction a month earlier. If he were allergic to strawberries I would have seen the same reaction. The difference between my strawberries and the ones he had in the restaurant were now obvious. Mine were organic.

I waited until later in the day before addressing this new information. I wanted to be sure there was no delayed reaction. "Josh, you ate strawberries today and you didn't cry." For a moment he was taken aback and I could tell he was searching his brain for an explanation. "I don't think you are allergic to strawberries at all. I think you are allergic to strawberries that are not organic."

In that moment, Joshua felt a sense of freedom. He was free to eat strawberries as long as they were free of chemicals. He loved his strawberry patch and he spent many hours feasting in it over the next few weeks without any reaction.

From that experience, we learned to buy only strawberries that were organically grown and pesticide free. It's important to note here that we also learned to be wary of products made with strawberries. If strawberries were listed as an ingredient on a label, they needed to be organic as well or Joshua could have a reaction.

I always laugh about the fact that Joshua was an expensive child. The truth was, I was happy to invest our money in making sure he was happy and healthy. I believe we spent our money wisely. I was less concerned about our lack of health insurance coverage. The good food we ate was our medicine and the changes we made in our environment were a greater and far less-expensive health insurance policy. I never felt cheated when investing in these types of practices.

Organic As a Way of Life

It was becoming clear to me that there was an undeniable relationship between food intake and behavior. The difference in Joshua's behavior between organic and conventional food was obvious at times and not so obvious at other times. I was always conscious of watching for changes to pinpoint the major culprits. Joshua became my full-time job.

Certain conventional foods, such as strawberries, invoked immediate responses; bananas were another one of those foods. After ingesting a conventional banana, Joshua would jump on the furniture and run rampant throughout the house. Immediately, organic bananas replaced conventional ones and Joshua's behavior noticeably changed.

Shortly thereafter I was reading a book by Dr. Bernard Jenson who stated that the worst sprayed fruits were strawberries, bananas and grapes (which would include raisins of course). Joshua had already confirmed two of these three fruits. Raisins and grapes were now added to my list of "organic only" foods. Each change I made allowed me to watch as Joshua's overall health continued to improve. It became common practice to avoid these three fruits or take organic ones with him wherever Joshua ventured. He was learning well that he was in charge of his overall health and happiness.

Joshua's health both physically and emotionally greatly improved when we replaced these particular fruits with the organic ones. I then began to wonder, could other non-organic foods be causing problems? Could other sprayed fruits be giving him a more subtle reaction? If they were affecting Joshua, were they also affecting all of us?

Owning a health food store allowed me to connect to organic distributors. I continued to fill our shelves with a vast assortment of organic products. We became an icon in the community teaching organic as a way of life and we were enjoying each step we took. We learned to eat what was in season. Though our diets were limited, the food we ate was cleaner and healthier than the non-organic alternatives.

The more I cooked with organic ingredients, the better the effect on Joshua. His attitude was changing before our eyes. His mood swings were becoming nonexistent. He was emotionally happier and more content. He was enjoying this newfound freedom of feeling joy within himself.

Joshua was never subjected to any form of medication during his early years. Instead, he was provided a steady diet of whole grains, fresh organic fruits and vegetables, nuts, seeds, and beans. His milk products were made from soy, rice, or from a goat; never a cow.

We were also blessed to have a well in our backyard that produced pure drinking water. If our water was anything less than pure, Joshua would have informed us immediately. Joshua drank an abundant supply of pure clean water. Soda was never on our menu.

We learned that it was not the quantity but the quality of food that was important to the well being of the body. Better quality food nourishes the body and the mind, and that's what we were trying to accomplish whenever we sat down together to have a meal.

Besides artificial colors and preservatives, sugars regularly played a huge role in affecting Joshua's health. White sugars caused hyperactivity. Joshua did very well when using pure maple syrup and organic blue agave as alternatives to refined sugars. Small amounts of cane juice crystals or raw cane sugar proved acceptable for parties, but pure maple syrup and agaves never caused a reaction. Pure maple syrup is an acceptable substitute in any recipe that calls for sugar. I learned this simple formula:

For every cup of white sugar, substitute 2/3 cup of pure maple syrup. Additional dry ingredients may need to be added to compensate for the liquid ingredients contained in the maple syrup.

When I add up the cost of the types of food and the amounts of those foods required to keep Joshua happy, the obvious conclusion is that our son cost us a small fortune. He was worth every penny we spent on him and ultimately on us. Eating the best quality food became a way of life for our entire family.

Home Away

As Joshua naturally ventured further from home, I made a conscious effort to watch for changes to his health and personality. He was developing a social life away from us. This simultaneously excited and concerned me. I wanted to remain aware of any changes that might take place as more choices were afforded him from the outside world.

His friends' homes introduced Joshua to a world that up-to-now had been off-limits and foreign to him, the world of fast food laced with chemicals. One day, Joshua came home from a friend's house and shared his experience with me.

"Mom, people don't cook at their homes. They don't eat real food."
He found himself in the presence of microwaves, frozen foods and
packaged products. He did not like what he was seeing and he did not
want to eat food prepared using any of these foreign methods. When
friends' families offered him something to eat, he would politely decline.
When the issue was pushed, he knew to explain, "I'm allergic to that
food. It's okay. I'll eat when I get home." Joshua learned to be the
supreme diplomat.

The result of all this polite declining, however, was that Joshua would be starving by the time he arrived home. I learned to have a meal ready upon his return. He appreciated the time we took to prepare his fresh, organic food.

He also began to understand the importance of having a family who thought he was worthy of their time and effort. It took a while, but Joshua finally found a friend whose family somewhat resembled his own.

One of his best friends (then and now) was Brian. Joshua loved
going to Brian's house, primarily because Brian's family was different.
Brian's mom loved to cook and she cooked with real food. Her dinners
were filled with fresh vegetables, grains and meats, and she often
prepared a chicken dish just for Joshua. Her cooking reminded Joshua
of home. Though he realized she was not using organic ingredients, the
vegetables were always fresh and he felt safe sharing a meal with his
new family.

This was an especially happy time for Joshua. He was stepping out
of his safety net to explore the world, and perhaps to discover who he
was and who he wanted to be. He was learning to create relationships
that allowed him to expand his horizons and ushered him away from his
home. He felt connected to Brian's family, and he continued to spend

more time with them. Eventually, we saw little of Joshua on the weekends. He was growing up, and that was good.

I was ecstatic about this latest chain of events, particularly since Brian's family was involved in Joshua's growth. This scenario held promise that Joshua could spend time with his friends without getting physically ill. He learned his lessons well and was now using that knowledge to stay healthy in the real world. He was very aware of the conventional foods that caused a reaction such as strawberries, grapes and bananas; and he was not afraid to omit them from his plate. Life was finally looking more "normal" in many respects. Joshua was taking care of his own needs; and he was learning to keep himself safe wherever he went.

It was shortly thereafter, however, that I began to notice emotional shifts in his behavior. These shifts occurred after he spent a weekend away at Brian's house. He would leave our home happy and excited and return angry and intolerant. His anger was often channeled directly at me.

I saw a pattern developing, and I was not sure how to approach it. I watched his behavior for a few more weekends to confirm my suspicions before I decided to address the situation. It became evident to me that, although his physical body seemed unaffected, his emotional body was in a state of turmoil.

Although he was not coming home with rashes, swollen glands or headaches, he was definitely coming home with an attitude. "How do I approach Joshua with these observations?" My opportunity came soon enough.

One weekend, Brian and his family went away on vacation. It was the first time in a long time that Joshua was forced to stay home with us. I enjoyed his company. Throughout the weekend, he was balanced and happy. I waited until the end of the weekend to share my thoughts with him.

"Joshua, I've been watching you each time you come home after spending a weekend with Brian. I know you feel good physically, but I think the food you are eating is affecting you emotionally. You come

home angry. You lash out at me and I don't know what to do about this."

His shields immediately went up. Joshua did not want to hear my concerns. Perhaps he was afraid of where this conversation might be headed. He had no intention of giving up his second family he had come to love so much. Nor did he wish to entertain any suggestions that might restrict him from them. I truly did not want that to happen either. I decided to let my words sit with him for a while. I planted a seed and I needed to allow that seed to grow where it may.

The following weekend, Joshua asked to sleep over Brian's home. I said yes, of course. It was a reasonable request that I would never deny him. So off he went, happy to be back in the company of his best friend. When he returned home the next day, he was angry at me again. "Okay," I thought. "Now is a good time to deal with this."

We sat down for a serious heart-to-heart talk. "Joshua, why are you so angry at me? There's really no reason for it. It's obvious to me that you come back from Brian's feeling intolerant. I just want to help you understand what may be affecting you in this way."

This time Joshua did not deny the truth. He recognized his anger and freely admitted this to me. I was proud of him for taking that important step. He clearly did not want to be that angry person. He liked getting along with everyone. He knew he had decisions to make. This presented another opportunity to solve a problem for himself.

Joshua loved Brian and his family and he loved being at their house. He needed to address this problem in his own way. He started by paying closer attention to the foods he ate while there, and learned how to feel oncoming emotional shifts in their early stages. He became increasingly aware of the types of food that brought on a reaction and the types of food that did not. Any food he determined to be problematic was quickly replaced with a similar food from home.

It became obvious that refined sugars and carbohydrates in cereal and bread products were causing issues for him. Weekends at Brian's house now included packing clothes and pillows, blankets and food. Joshua's backpack was always filled with whole grain cereals, organic sprouted breads and bagels as well as organic bananas and soy milk. If he had nothing else to eat, he could survive on his favorite staple foods.

Joshua was developing a keen rhythm with an entirely new aspect of his body language and he enjoyed the learning experience. He connected with his body the moment a shift occurred and understood what each shift was telling him. He realized that to avoid the same problems in the future, he had to learn which foods were tied to his emotional reactions.

Brian's mom was gracious about the whole situation. She encouraged Joshua to do whatever was necessary to stay healthy and remain a part of their family. Brian's family loved Joshua and wanted to ensure he could continue his weekly visits.

It wasn't easy for a child to admit his differences; even more difficult to have to deal with those differences by himself. For Joshua it was worth the effort.

When all was said and done, Joshua was ultimately responsible for his physical and emotional health. He was learning the meaning of strength and determination, and the importance of speaking his truth and honoring his own needs. He was also learning to surround himself with friends who loved and supported him. Brian was one of those friends.

Food to Go

Although Joshua was comfortable packing food at Brian's house, he did not always feel as comfortable doing the same at other places he ventured. Friends, neighbors and even some family members had a hard time understanding why Joshua consistently refused to eat at their homes. He was not trying to be rude; he was just trying to stay healthy. There were instances when Joshua was unable to eat anything that was offered. I learned to have food ready and waiting when he returned. His quest to feed his hunger was akin to watching a shark in a feeding frenzy.

By the time he entered his early teens, he was growing tired of the hunger game. "Why don't you bring food with you when you visit your friends? It could solve your hunger problem." Joshua felt uncomfortable. He felt weird already and the thought of bringing weird food to his friends made him even more uncomfortable. I thought it silly. Our food was not weird. It was simply organic, whole grain and healthy, the way food should be. I did not push the issue. I allowed him to think about our conversation, hoping he would find a solution to another problem.

It did not take long before Joshua changed his mind. "I think I want to start taking food with me. I am always hungry and sometimes I have to come home before I really want to. What should I take?" That was a good question.

"Let's think about what is easy and filling." I suggested he begin with things that he could handle himself: sprouted bagels and breads; almond butter; organic jellies; cereals and soy milk. That felt good to him. He could make everything himself, it would fill him up and he did not have to ask anyone to do anything special for him. That was always a concern. He did not want to create added work or responsibility for his friends' parents. It was settled. Joshua was going to meet his own needs so he could be with friends.

Once began, Joshua became very comfortable packing food wherever he went. The embarrassment he first felt was gone. Friends and parents grew accustomed to Joshua's need to bring his own food to their homes, most of which was all new to their world. His "food to go" was a natural progression of Joshua's lifestyle. As time went on, he never left home without a huge parcel in his backpack. The food became something of a novelty and Joshua enjoyed sharing it with his friends and their families.

Joshua made plans to stay over at Justin's house one evening. Justin lived up the street from us. The two had been good friends for a long time, and Justin's family had come to terms with our strange ways.

Before leaving, Joshua filled a shopping bag with his favorite food, the usual staples of his diet. Joshua could survive forever on whole grains and nut butters, especially when adding a bowl of whole grain cereal and soy milk to the mix.

Joshua's backpack was filled. I expected a phone call that he would be staying extra days. I found myself wondering if he truly miscalculated or whether he had a clear goal in mind. My thought was later confirmed. When he arrived home, I found his backpack empty of any leftovers. "You ate all that food?" I inquired with a surprised voice. Normally what was not consumed was returned for later use.

"No, there was a bunch left over. Justin's mom liked the bagels and the almond butter; I left the rest so they could enjoy them." Now wasn't that an interesting turn of events. They enjoyed Joshua's food!

What a wonderful shift of energy. Joshua turned a once embarrassing moment into a proud moment. He was teaching people that there was a variety of great food out there waiting to be tasted.

A week later, Justin's mom came into our store. "Where are those bagels and almond butter that Joshua left at our house last week? I want to buy some. They are really good!" Before walking out the door, she left a clear message for my son. "Please tell Joshua he is welcome to bring samples to our house anytime!"

Chapter Six

~ The School Years ~

Joshua was faced with chemicals everywhere. School was no exception. It was often a source of chemical poisoning that had severe affects. His ability to learn and focus was often compromised. Sometimes school was not safe for Joshua to attend.

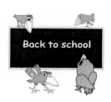

Joshua was in first grade; it was early November. Joshua liked school and he liked to learn. He still does. Things were going well, until one day when he arrived home disoriented and light headed. Within hours his eyes were irritated and he was having problems breathing. "Mom, the gymnasium smells really bad. I think they put something on the floor. I can't breathe when I go into the gym." Polyurethane filled my mind.

The following day, I called the office to confirm my suspicions. "The gym floor had urethane applied to it over the weekend while the children were away. It is normal maintenance." I knew this was not going to be good for Joshua. How could it be good for any child? I decided to visit the school to see just how bad it was.

Before I got to the gymnasium, the smell of urethane permeated the main corridor. It was so intense, it turned my stomach. As I looked around, the staff seemed unaffected. Could they be pretending this smell was normal? Were they really oblivious to this awful odor? Was this chemical affecting other children?

I peeked inside the doors. A group of little people were running up and down the gymnasium floor inhaling toxic fumes. Could this be healthy for these little bodies? Was anyone thinking at all? Could the fumes have already affected their brains?

    I refocused my thoughts back to Joshua; my main concern was his health at the moment. I immediately requested a meeting with the principal.

This was not my first meeting; it would not be my last. She was fully aware of Joshua's reactions, and a request for a meeting meant Joshua was reacting. I was an involved mother, maybe too involved for their liking. I tried to be understanding of their position when it came to chemicals. In turn, they tried to be understanding of Joshua.

    "Joshua came home sick yesterday. He is having difficulty breathing. The urethane on the gymnasium floor is making him ill. There is no way he will be able to go into that gymnasium until the smell dissipates."

    "Joshua can't miss gym class. It is required that he take it." She was worried about Joshua missing gym class; I was concerned that gym class could kill him! Joshua was excused from gym class.

    The first few days that he was excused from gym, he experienced minor improvement. As the week progressed, his inability to breathe worsened. When he was home on weekends his body had the opportunity to heal and his symptoms subsided. By the middle of the second week, they returned with a vengeance. Joshua realized the problem. "I have to walk past the gym to get to the cafeteria and the smell still bothers me." Here was a problem that needed a solution.

    "Would it be better to have your lunch in your classroom?" Joshua always brought his lunch so he did not really need to go to the cafeteria.

    That did not suit him at all. "I like being with my friends in the cafeteria. I don't want to eat lunch alone. That's not fair!" Joshua was right. He had every right to socialize with his friends at lunchtime. There had to be another solution. We would have to find it.

By evening, Joshua came downstairs with a proposal, "I think I can avoid the gym completely if I go out the side door near my classroom and walk around the school right into the cafeteria by the front door."

"Is that something you would be comfortable doing?" I asked with concern. It seemed extreme; yet he did not have another solution that he felt would work. By now Joshua was known to be weird among the administration, the teachers and his peers. He was used to doing things differently. It was just another precaution to ensure his health.

"I just want to be able to eat in the cafeteria, Mom." It was settled. I would go to school in the morning to help Joshua speak his case. Joshua and I were in charge of his school environment. We were good at finding solutions to problems; all we needed was the school's support. I always approached them with concern and determination for Joshua's right to be healthy.

The staff was learning to work with us. They did not want Joshua to be ill either. Joshua was a kind and likable child. They wanted to help us through this ordeal. They just didn't understand it.

I made a date to visit the school the following morning. By the time I arrived, Joshua had already worked out his plan with his teacher. He took us both to the side door that led out to the school yard. We walked through his plan.

His teacher was completely agreeable. "Joshua is a good boy. I trust that he is responsible enough to do this. Are you okay with him walking outside the school to get to the cafeteria?" If Joshua felt safe, I felt safe too.

Within a few short days he knew his plan was working. He was able to breathe and think clearly again. By the end of the week, his symptoms disappeared all together. Missing gym class for a month was the healthiest choice.

Teaching the Staff

It concerned me that the school believed Joshua was unique to chemical sensitivities. It concerned me more that parents were unaware of how chemicals may be affecting their own children. Chemicals of this nature clogged Joshua's system to the point he could not think or focus in school. As he grew, he realized immediately that this was a symptom of chemical poisoning. With so many issues relating to a child's inability to think or focus today, should we be looking at chemical sensitivities to help deal with some of these problems?

I felt compelled to speak to those in power to see if I could help create change, not only for Joshua, but for other children who may unknowingly be affected as well. When I called the office, I was directed to the assistant principal to address my concerns. I made an appointment for the following day.

I wondered what I would face when I arrived. My experience had taught me that many people are defensive about their ability to use chemicals whenever and wherever they deem necessary. I did not want to demand a solution; I simply wanted to open a doorway for discussion. What I saw once I arrived at her office amazed me.

The assistant principal's room was cold. It was a blustery day and yet her window was wide opened. "That's strange," I thought to myself. On her desk was a huge box of Kleenex tissue that she was repeatedly using to blow her nose. She looked awful. Her mucus membranes were stuffed up and her eyes looked swollen. She appeared to have the same symptoms as Joshua.

I refocused myself. I was there on my own business; not hers. I began to voice my concerns. "Joshua is very affected by the urethane smell in the gym and the halls. He can't even walk by it without becoming ill. We worked out a solution; however, I am still concerned how it might be affecting other children. I think it is unhealthy that we allow children to run up and down the gymnasium breathing in these toxic fumes."

She continued to sneeze and blow her nose with coughing fits in between. When she was able to get her composure back, her answer took me by surprise, "Oh, I definitely think it's a problem. I've been sick since the floor was done. I know the urethane is making me ill!" She had great sympathy for Joshua's sensitivities. She understood them completely. Incidentally, her office was directly across from the gymnasium.

It boggled my mind. She knew that the gym was making her ill and yet, she was resigned to the fact that she had to live with it. "Isn't there something that can be done? Why can't we do this type of work during the summer months when the school is empty?" She thought that was a great idea, yet I did not feel that she would take on the challenge.

Why wouldn't she fight for her right to be healthy? Did she feel she had no right to demand a safe environment? How many other children were being affected by urethanes? I could not be complacent. Not only did Joshua deserve better; every person in the building deserved better. Someone had to address this. I realized that someone was me.

Teaching the Board

I attended the next Board of Education meeting, ready and willing to inform the members of the error of their ways. After bringing them up to date with Joshua's dilemma and his solutions to his problem as well as my visit with the assistant principal, I now had a list of questions I wanted addressed:

-Why did we urethane the gym floors during the school year?
-Why could we not urethane them during the summer months?
-Why were we not using less toxic latex polyurethanes?
-If Joshua was ill from this chemical, were other children affected?
-Do these chemicals affect a child's ability to think and learn?

"We have been dealing with Joshua's chemical sensitivities since he was very little. One thing Joshua is certain about is that when he is poisoned by a chemical, it affects his ability to think which in turn affects his ability to learn to his fullest potential."

I had an attentive audience. They listened; heads were nodding in agreement. Some of the Board members began wondering the same things. I thought I saw a light at the end of this tunnel.

I am not aware of the policies at the school presently; however, I do know that the policies were modified for as long as Joshua was in elementary school. Oil based urethanes were replaced with less toxic latex urethanes, and every effort was made to do this type of work during the summer months. However, the changes were implemented at the elementary school only. Each time Joshua graduated to a new school, the problem followed, and we were forced to deal with each school individually.

The Great Paper Chase

It seemed that each new grade unleashed a new allergy. Fifth grade was challenging. One day Joshua came home from school swollen. Hives were rampant and roamed over his entire body. This incident was particularly confusing, as it took time to find the source:

The hives were relentless, especially at night. Joshua was kept awake with an intense itching that appeared and disappeared from one part of his body to another. His condition worsened as the week continued and often his hands looked swollen. By Friday, I was very concerned. "Joshua, stay home today. I will call your teacher and pick up your homework so you don't get behind." He desperately agreed. Saturday the hives still plagued him, but to a much lesser extent and by Sunday morning he was hive free. He was happy to feel normal again.

Monday he was back at school and by Monday night the hives reappeared. Now we were sure the problem was coming from inside the school. We just didn't know where. "What about science or art class? Did you start a new project?" We learned by now that the chemicals used in both classes could create havoc with Joshua's system that he often had to avoid; however, he was sure that was not the problem.

What was the problem then? We talked about unusual smells that might be provoking his senses. Joshua had no answers. Again, by the end of the weekend the symptoms improved. We hoped with time the cause would be revealed.

By the third week Joshua was frustrated. I continued to keep him home on Fridays to give his body a chance to recover; by Sunday morning he felt relief.

Missing school had its disadvantages. Joshua always had pages of school work to make up. This particular weekend was busy, so Joshua was behind. We agreed that after dinner on Sunday, he would have to get it all done. He went to his room immediately after dinner and took out his books, paper and pencils. Within minutes, he ran down the stairs yelling with excitement, "Mom, I figured out the problem. It's the yellow paper! When I got upstairs I pulled the yellow paper out of my book bag and my nose stuffed up immediately!"

Yellow lined paper was used at school for many of his assignments. Was the mystery finally solved? "Stop using the yellow paper. We will deal with this in the morning."

By morning, his hands were swollen to twice their size and he was very itchy. I took him to school and asked to see the principal. Joshua sat next to me with his swollen hands. The principal sat and listened to the entire story and how we came upon the fact that the yellow paper was the cause of Joshua's hulk sized hands. He listened with little emotion, and I was quite sure he did not believe any of it. However, that was not my concern. Joshua and I knew for certain that the yellow paper had to go.

"What Joshua needs is to make sure he does not have to touch yellow paper again." The principal assured me that he would communicate this problem to Joshua's teacher so he could avoid the problem in the future.

Joshua came home that day very upset. "My teacher put a yellow paper on my desk when he handed out our assignment. I wouldn't touch it, Mom." Joshua was not stupid. He knew what would happen if he touched that yellow paper.

"What did you do?" I asked. He told me that he stared at it for a while trying to decide what his next move should be. He decided his pencil was his best defense. With a swoop of his eraser on the end of his pencil, he pushed the yellow paper off his desk and onto the floor. I can only imagine the look on the teacher's face.

The teacher warned Joshua, "Don't do that again." Joshua tried to explain to his teacher the reason for his actions, but the teacher did not understand the seriousness of the situation. Why should he? If it was that serious, he would have been informed by someone other than a small boy.

Joshua had every right to be upset. I was upset too. It seemed we were getting no help from the school. I called the principal immediately. After I explained what happened to Joshua at school, he described what transpired in his office after we left. "I put a note in his teacher's box. If he already picked up his mail, he may not get it until tomorrow morning. He probably isn't aware of the situation yet."

Was he serious? Did he think a letter that may not be read until the next day was a solution to Joshua's swollen hands? I was enraged. The only ones taking this situation seriously were me and Joshua.

Truthfully, I was angry with myself that I did not address the problem directly with Joshua's teacher. We were learning that going right to the source was our best option. Why did I even get the principal involved? I called the teacher and explained the situation. He was very understanding. Joshua was excused from yellow paper.

Every Day is Earth Day

At that particular time, the school was recycling only white paper. The world was learning the importance of recycling, and white paper was at the forefront of the effort. Yellow paper was thrown out in the trash.

It so happened that I was appointed Earth Day Coordinator for our town that year. I was asked to speak to the sixth grade class on environmental issues of concern to the community. It was a perfect forum to share Joshua's experience with a compassionate audience.

After sharing Joshua's experience with the yellow paper and hives. I asked, "Why does the school continue to use yellow paper when it is not recyclable? Doesn't it make sense to use paper that we can recycle and reuse? What kind of example was the school setting for others?"

The students listened intently. They took the information they received at our meeting and went into action. They were able to do that which I could not; they voiced their concerns to the principal and he listened. Shortly afterwards, yellow paper was no longer used in the school system. All paper was white and recycled. Change was good!

Chapter Seven

~ Playground of Poisons ~

Joshua had been a conduit for change at his other schools, and those changes served him well. He entered high school confident that he would continue to teach others the importance of a healthy environment.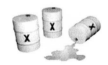

It was late September of Joshua's freshman year. "My friends are playing football at the high school this afternoon. Can you give me a ride?" It was great to see him adjusting so well into high school life. He was healthy and happy. I dropped him off with instructions to pick him up at 4:30. By the time I arrived, the expression on his face told me how much fun he had, until...

As I backed the car out of our parking space, I noticed a small 3"x5" sign attached to the metal fence. Joshua noticed it at the same time. We did not have to say a word. We each knew what the sign said: "Pesticide Application." Why had we not noticed it when I dropped him off? It was mandated that a warning be posted, however, it was not mandated that it be big enough to be noticed. I was not happy; neither was Joshua. Had we seen it earlier, he and his friends could have chosen to play on another field.

By evening, Joshua's breathing was labored, and each day became worse than the previous one. His head was foggy and he could not concentrate on his school work. By the fourth day, the symptoms began to subside as we knew they would. Time and patience were on his side.

When he returned home from school on Thursday, he was quite upset. "The first football game of the season is this Friday. I don't want to miss going to the game!" I knew he was afraid of the consequences.

"If you go back on that field you will probably make yourself sick again. I am not sure if a second exposure will be worse than the first. Are you willing to take that chance?"

"I can try to stay as far away from the field as possible. I can walk around the back of the bleachers and sit way up at the top. I want to go to the game, Mom." How could I argue? His first high school football game meant a lot to him. He felt strongly he wanted to be there.

At first it seemed the symptoms might be mild. The second day he was conscious of a reaction; however, he felt it may not be as severe as the previous one. He was happy he made the choice to go; however, as the days passed his symptoms worsened. By the time he went to school on Monday, he was coughing and had difficulty breathing. He began to question if he made the right decision. It took until Wednesday evening before he was feeling well again.

The second football game of the season was another home game. "I don't think I'm going to the game this week," he informed me. He was not ready for another round of illness and decided it best if he avoided the fields for a little while. The following week, the team was away which made him very happy. By month's end, he was back on the field with no ill effects whatsoever. This allowed us to understand how long he needed to avoid the chemical applications on the fields.

What I should do with this information was always a question I had to answer. I believed Joshua could not be the only child who was experiencing the effects of these chemicals. Other children might be having reactions and not realizing the field was the cause. I decided to share my information with the powers to be. I attended the next school board meeting.

Although I spoke at a school board meeting when he was much younger, this was a new group of members, and it would be the first they would hear of a student named Joshua. I wanted to be prepared.

The school board had the power to make changes that could help Joshua feel safe in school. I believed that is exactly what they would want to do.

Hear No Evil

A school board meeting can be very intimidating; however, I was serving my second term as a member of the town council, so I understood the procedures and how the hierarchy worked. My goal was to help everyone realize the importance of a chemical free school by attempting to get them to understand the seriousness of Joshua's situation. I also hoped they would think about the possibility the chemicals may be having on other children and their staff.

When it was time for public comment, I took my turn at the microphone. I began with a brief introduction of Joshua's experiences throughout his school years. I explained how chemicals manifest different symptoms in his body dependent upon the toxicity of the chemical. I was also clear that chemicals could affect his ability to think and learn and how they played havoc with his emotions.

I explained how he had to avoid the school fields to feel safe and healthy. I finished my presentation with one simple request, "I would like copies of the MSDS sheets of any chemical used on the school grounds. This will help me understand more clearly the side effects of each one and what exactly may be affecting Joshua." I was already aware that it was mandatory that MSDS sheets be made available upon request.

It took a little while and a few rounds of phone calls before my request was honored. I sat down one night and read each one. Before me was a list of Joshua's symptoms: Nausea, headaches, inability to concentrate, asthma, dizziness, skin rashes...

The list went on and on. I thought this fascinating. I wondered, "Has anyone with any authority read these sheets? Does anyone know about the chemicals we are subjecting our children to?"

Our children were not only allowed, but expected, to play on these fields almost immediately after chemical spraying. There was no concern or thought given to how anyone might be affected. I was sure this was just an oversight. I came to the conclusion that no one could have possibly read these sheets. Certainly they would want to know and be informed. Again, it was my job to teach them. I returned to the next school board meeting. I was certain they would embrace this information and be even more concerned than I was; or would they?

Energy is very powerful. We can't see it, but we certainly can feel it. From the moment I walked into that meeting, I felt like an unwelcome guest. I felt the members would have been relieved had I turned around and walked away. I felt they did not want to hear what I had to say. At that moment, I recognized the old saying, "See no evil; speak no evil; hear no evil." Oh darn, I was the "evil" they did not want to look at, speak to, or hear from. Now what?

I had a mission to accomplish. "Evil" was not leaving. I knew this was not going to be easy, but it had to be done. It was important that the message was spoken and I was the messenger. I took out the MSDS sheets and began to read from them, realizing no one had a clue what they contained. I felt the ice in the room gently begin to unfreeze. I had their attention for the moment and I took full advantage of it.

I scanned their faces and recognized a few allies among the group. I thought it best to focus on them, which kept my hands from trembling. Yes, group energy is very powerful. Their force of denial directed at me made me feel small and insignificant. I had to move beyond that force and into my power of truth.

I again shared Joshua's experiences on and off the fields. I compared the possible symptoms listed on the MSDS sheets with the symptoms Joshua experienced after being subjected to the sprayed fields. I asked if we as a community would consider looking at alternative ways to take care of our fields. I believed that Joshua had a right to play on those fields without fear. "I am very willing to look for organic alternatives to chemical applications. I would like to serve our community and I would like Joshua to be able to attend events on our school fields without fear of becoming ill."

There can be no discussion at a meeting unless it is specifically on the agenda. I was aware of this, so I did not expect a response. "I would like to request that the chemicals we use on our school fields be put on the next agenda so discussion may begin about the concerns I have presented." They granted me that wish.

I was back at the next meeting. I was beginning to become a regular. Again, that unwelcoming feeling permeated the room. It did not bother me quite as much as the previous month. Maybe I was getting used to it.

With little discussion, I was informed that the school board had no intention of changing the chemicals used on the fields. The chairperson stated the school board's position, "Killingly is noted for having some of the nicest fields in Northeast Connecticut. We are happy with the results the chemicals provide."

I had to get this straight in my mind. "Are you telling me that the quality of your fields take precedence over Joshua's education and health?" It seemed the majority of the members agreed with the chairperson. They may have agreed with him; I did not.

"You realize that this chemical may be the cause of Joshua's symptoms, and yet you feel it is okay to continue using it on our playing fields creating a playground of poisons?" That label did not go over well. I was now officially the enemy.

Killingly school system strived for "Excellence in Education." We posted this motto all over the school, advertised it in newspapers, and proudly announced it on letterheads, which is all well and good, unless it is not the truth. We can say anything we want; but it is what we do that is most important. Joshua felt he was being denied an excellent education under the present circumstances. I agreed with Joshua.

The First Concession

I continued to worry about other students. I knew children who experienced constant headaches, sore throats and asthma. I knew even more who had difficulty concentrating in school. Why was I the only one discussing the possibility that the fields might be a source of some of the same problems? "Hear no evil" was at the forefront right about now. Down went the gavel; discussion was closed. The fields would continue to be sprayed; however, I did get one small concession.

"What we will do, Mrs. Wojcik, is notify you and Joshua personally before each chemical application on the fields." At least they were giving us time to make decisions so Joshua could avoid the situation.

"Okay," I thought, "I guess that's better than nothing." But was it? I found out later that legally every parent has a right to be informed of pesticide spraying. That was interesting. I won a concession I had the right to all along.

The following spring, I received my personal letter informing me the dates the fields were scheduled to be sprayed. I made an appointment with the principal. "If you insist on poisoning the fields, Joshua will not be able to take gym class." It appeared no one had considered this as a possibility.

The principal replied adamantly, "Gym class is mandatory. Joshua has to take it."

"Not on those fields. There must be another option that he can do during that time inside the school. He will not be subjected to illness."

After much discussion, Joshua was excused from going on the fields for two weeks following each round of spraying. The principal was quite compassionate regarding the ordeal. It was he who suggested the weight room at the end of the gymnasium hallway. "The weight room is used by the wrestling team for work outs. Joshua can use it to avoid the fields. He will be getting the required exercise so I will approve it in place of his gym class."

Joshua was ecstatic. Weight training had always been a dream and here it was being offered to him for free! Angels work in unusual ways. For two weeks each day, Joshua got off the bus and went directly into the school. During gym period, he was left alone in the weight room and it suited him well!

As time progressed, however, Joshua felt isolated from his friends. His frustration increased along with his sensitivity levels. I was beginning to see a direct correlation between his symptoms and his emotions. However, I did not know how to help him heal his emotions. I understood his frustration; no one cared. His body was reacting to his pain.

The fields were sprayed during weekends when the children were not at school. That was a good decision. One Monday, after the fields had been sprayed, the weather turned warm and windy. The windows of the school were wide opened and Joshua had a few classes in rooms facing the soccer field. By Thursday of that week, he felt school was making him ill again. He came home that afternoon with a sore throat.

By evening, his throat was closing, making it difficult to breathe. I kept him home on Friday, and with the help of his constitutional homeopathic remedy, he felt better throughout the day.

Then we witnessed an even more interesting event. Holly Beth got off the bus that afternoon. Upon entering the house, she sat down next to her brother to share her day with him. Immediately he began to sneeze uncontrollably. That put the icing on the cake. He was now allergic to his sister! I surmised she was carrying the chemical in her clothing and Joshua was instantly reacting. I was ready to put him in a bubble.

When he returned to school the following week, the symptoms were less severe. He was able to make it through the whole week without missing any school, a feat in itself. The third week he was symptom free.

Again, I felt the need to report Joshua's experiences to the school board. This time I decided to write a letter. The letter clearly stated that Joshua's system was becoming more sensitive with each spraying.

I insisted on a solution so Joshua could be healthy at school. Either the spraying had to stop or Joshua had to stop going to school. By mid summer, we received our official notification for the fall schedule.

Joshua was totally frustrated. "They really won't stop spraying the fields so I can go to school?" I couldn't believe it either.

"You and I have to decide how to keep you healthy." We discussed the options. We came to the conclusion that for Joshua to be healthy, he had to avoid the school all together following each application. I brought our proposal to the principal. It was easy to understand.

"For the first week after each spraying, Joshua will be allowed to stay at home. I will pick up his homework each day, and he will commit to keep up with his school work. He will try to return to school during the second week. Joshua will have final say dependent upon his body's reactions."

I must interject here. Imagine a child since kindergarten who packed his lunches to take to school and to his friends' homes. Picture a child who suffered in a home using chemical cleaners. This was also a child who kept bottled water at his side before it was a fashion statement. With all his weirdness and all his issues, he was loved by all his friends. Joshua had great friends. They watched out for him and were on constant alert should a chemical invade his space. They accepted him with all his differences.

The Spraying Never Stops

Joshua's sophomore year was a repeat performance of his freshman year. During the fall months, he missed many weeks of school. Winter came and went and by early spring, we received another official letter notifying us that the fields would be sprayed in the spring and fall. I did not know how much more either of us could take. Joshua was frustrated; I was disgusted. I began to wonder, "Who is responsible to ensure this child receives an education?" No one dared come forward. It seemed acceptable with the administration that Joshua spent more time out of school than in it.

One of the spring sprayings was scheduled for June 7, obviously without any thought attached to it. I say this because the first day of summer vacation was June 18. Joshua read the letter and could not contain himself. "Why can't they wait to spray the fields until after June 18? If they spray on June 7, I won't be able to finish out the school year." The only one making any sense at that moment was Joshua.

I approached the assistant superintendent with Joshua's concern. He listened and after a few moments, he agreed. He wondered out loud why anyone would consider spraying the fields before summer vacation. I felt he was beginning to think it was not such a good idea either. He promised to look into it and call us in the morning. I passed this information on to Joshua. He felt empowered for the first time in a very long time. He was learning to voice his opinions without fear.

I was not home when the assistant superintendent called the following day. Joshua answered the phone giving the two of them an opportunity to speak to one another directly. For the first time, Joshua was a voice behind the issue. He was not a figment of my imagination. He was a real person with legitimate concerns.

Joshua had an opportunity to speak his feelings. The assistant superintendent listened. "I promise Joshua that the fields will not be sprayed while school is in session. We made a decision to wait until summer vacation." This personal contact set the stage for movement in a new direction.

This experience allowed Joshua to think about all the things he had gone through the past year. When I arrived home that afternoon he shared his conversation with me. He then turned and said, "Maybe no one really gets the flu or a cold at all, Mom. Maybe we are all being poisoned but we don't know it."

What could I say? "You might be right, Josh."

Is Anybody Listening?

Shortly after school ended, Joshua voiced his frustration.

"You know, Mom, I'm not going to be able to go to any football games this year if they spray the fields in September and October." My heart ached for him. Here he was in high school, unable to participate in any outdoor activities. All he wanted was to be able to go to school, and his request was consistently denied. That was enough for me. Was it enough for Joshua?

"Josh," I explained, "I believe you have a right to be in school. I believe that you are more important than the poisons they spray on the fields, but I need your help. I want to contact a newspaper and see if I can get your story out. Are you willing to go all the way with this? This is not about me, it's about you. Those in charge are not taking this seriously. Are you willing to speak to a reporter?"

I knew instantly how scared that thought made him feel. We were opening Pandora's Box and once opened it could not be shut. Whatever was in that box would be revealed for everyone to dissect. Was he willing to be dissected? Could he hold his power against an entire establishment that believed otherwise? Was he ready to fight for his health? He looked at me with concern, deep concern and said, "Okay Mom. I'll do whatever it takes. I want to be in school."

I was proud of him. He was choosing to step out of his box and share himself with the entire region. He was about to reveal how different he was.

I approached the superintendent before putting our next plan into action. I gave him an update on Joshua's concerns and his reactions up to this point. I also informed him that we were ready to fight for his right to be healthy both in the school and on the school grounds. There was little reaction from him. The fields continued to be more important.

I called the local newspapers to see if there was interest in his story. One newspaper decided to write about Joshua's experiences. We made an appointment for them to meet Joshua at the house. After the interview the reporter asked, "Can we go to the school to take pictures of you near the fields?" Joshua was aware that the fields had been recently sprayed. He reluctantly agreed. He did not like going anywhere near them, but he knew it was something he had to do.

The 3x5 warning sign had been prominently displayed on the fence near the entrance to the field. Seeing the sign made Joshua cringe. He held his breath (literally) as pictures were snapped with the sign in view. It was not a pretty picture.

We went back to the house and the interview continued. They talked about his experiences, his reactions, the MSDS sheets. She wanted to know how it felt not being able to attend school and to be isolated from his friends. He spoke honestly and candidly about his thoughts, his feelings and his experiences.

She wanted to know if there was anyone else she could contact to get a clearer picture from a medical point of view. We supplied her with Dr. Bill's name and number.

She called Dr. Bill, Joshua's homeopathic physician. He was happy to share his experiences with Joshua and other children who had these types of sensitivities. Dr. Bill explained what he felt was happening using an analogy:

> *"Children like Joshua are comparable to the canaries the old miners used to take down in the mines with them. Canaries are very fragile birds, and when the canary died, the miners knew they could no longer stay in the mines without being poisoned."*

I had not thought of it that way, but it was a perfect analogy. Our family learned to use Joshua in the same way. If a chemical made him ill, it was a warning for the rest of us.

The leaders of our community, however, did not feel the same. They did not think of Joshua as the yellow canary. They refused to believe that poisons could affect anyone. His warnings became a thorn in their sides. I felt sad for them, but I understood. How could they know any different?

The reporter also contacted an allergist at the local hospital who backed up Joshua's story. He had experience with chemically sensitive children and confirmed much of what we were saying. I never met this allergist, but he did comment that watching and being aware of what made Joshua sick was the only way to help him heal.

The article spurred much interest among people near and far. The issue was no longer about Joshua but about the future of how to make our schools safer for our children, all our children. The issue was about letting go of the fear that kept us from making healthy changes for the betterment of all in the community, including Joshua.

At our store, customers praised Joshua's efforts. They admired his determination. Shortly thereafter, a customer came into the store with a dilemma about her own son.

"Ryan developed a sore throat a few days ago. Later that day it turned into a full blown cough and now he is having trouble breathing. Joshua's story in the newspaper seems very similar to what Ryan is experiencing."

My first question was, "When did the symptoms begin?"

Her answer was no surprise to me, "His symptoms began immediately after playing golf at a local golf course." Was it a coincidence? At least Ryan's mother was thinking about the possibilities. Awareness is the first step toward healing.

Where Do We Go From Here?

We were always personally warned before each monthly spraying. It was August and Joshua was getting ready for his junior year. Our personal letter arrived stating that the fields would be sprayed in September.

Joshua was extremely upset. He did not understand why his concerns were not being addressed. He could not help but ask, "Why doesn't the school board take my problems seriously?"

I assured him, "Every great battle takes time to win. I'll never give up on your right to be in school. I hope you don't either." Joshua chose to remain at home the first week after the spraying while I arranged a meeting with the principal to discuss his future with gym upon his return. Again, Joshua was allowed to work out in the weight room so as not to lose his gym credits.

Tuesday evening after returning to school, the headaches and sore throat reappeared. Two of his classes faced the fields and the windows were wide open. We gave him his constitutional remedy, and it seemed to diminish the effects quickly. That was a good sign. He wanted to stay in school. Since his throat did not swell this time, he made the decision to live with these minor symptoms.

Being able to stay in school during this time allowed him to watch what was happening around him. He shared with me what he witnessed that week, "Mom," he said. "I sat in class the other day and watched the other kids. Some of them were coughing, others were sneezing. A group of them were constantly blowing their noses. Maybe I'm not the only one allergic to those fields. Maybe I'm just the only one who knows it."

I had to smile. I could not agree with him more. Until other parents considered the possibility, there was nothing we could do but continue to fight for his right to be healthy. Recognizing these symptoms in others, however, made Joshua realize that maybe he was not so different after all. Maybe he had the power to see differently. He was starting to appreciate his gift of conscious awareness.

I always felt fortunate to have a huge selection of alternative therapies to help Joshua heal. There were many modalities at our disposal. I studied them all. Joshua and I experimented together what helped and what didn't.

Being a part of the alternative healing world brought an assortment of healing therapies to our doorstep. I can't imagine what life would have been like without them.

The Painted Lockers

Winter finally arrived. The spraying stopped and Joshua was just getting back to feeling healthy again. He felt safe at school and was enjoying his freedom to roam without fear. This feeling of safety came to a quick halt. One December afternoon, he came home with the news.

"They painted the lockers in the upstairs hallway at school. The smell is so bad. There's no way I'll be able to handle it. I couldn't focus all afternoon. My mind was like a fog!" He spent the afternoon worried that his feeling of safety had just come to an abrupt end. "Why do these people have the need to poison me?"

I tried to assure him it was not intentionally. "They really don't know any better. They don't have a clue how serious it is to subject children to these chemicals." His frustration soared. I listened but my mind was racing trying to figure out what to do next. I did not want him to miss another day of school and neither did he.

"Is there any way you can avoid that area of the school?" He said he would try. He stayed as far away as possible, but this was more toxic than his body could handle. The paint was oil based, and it smelled horrible!

After a few days, a rash appeared under his arms and his glands swelled. His eyes watered and his skin itched. By the end of the week his face broke out in huge cysts; he was a mess. He pleaded for help, "Mom, what do I do?"

"Stay home tomorrow. I will go to the school and pick up your books. It will give me a chance to see exactly how bad it is."

I walked into the upstairs hall and the smell hit me in the face. The odor from the toxicity of this paint permeated the entire hallway. Children and teachers walked among these smells as if it were normal.

Was I the only one who thought this crazy? Could I really be wrong in thinking this was not healthy for any of them? No, I was not crazy. Expecting children to learn who are chemically poisoned is crazy.

The principal and I were on a first name basis by now. I voiced my concerns again. He listened. "Joshua's condition is worsening with each day. He needs a break from school. I'm going to keep him home until his body has time to discharge all these chemicals. I'll pick up his homework every day" (yet again). I could not contain myself and continued, "Certainly you don't plan to paint any more lockers while the children are trying to learn here? These chemicals affect Joshua's ability to learn; I can't believe it doesn't affect others. May I also ask, why are you painting in the middle of the school year and why in December when it's too cold to open windows for ventilation?"

I'm not sure if they were just tired of listening to me or if they were beginning to understand the seriousness of the situation. Whatever it was, the painting stopped and the windows were opened. It took weeks, but eventually, Joshua felt healthy enough to return to school. The rash under his arms disappeared, his energy level improved, and his face cleared up. Again, his school was safe. How long would it last?

Round and Round We Go

Spring of his junior year arrived with another letter. We were informed that the fields would be sprayed on April 18. Joshua was not ready to go through this ordeal again. He was feeling healthy; he wanted to stay healthy. Together, we made the decision to keep Joshua out of school the first week after the spraying took place to diminish his exposure levels. I collected his homework each day and he continued to feel healthy at home. He enjoyed being healthy; he missed being at school.

Joshua returned to school on April 27. He arrived home with a rash under his arms. By evening, his glands swelled. By the next morning his

95

eyes were small slits and his skin began breaking out in cysts. It was undeniable. The school poisoned him again. He was done; he had enough.

I set up a meeting with the superintendent. He was aware of the history. He knew the story. I got right to the point. "Joshua is done. He will not be subjected to any more sprayings, any more painting, or any more chemicals. He has a right to be healthy. If you won't allow him a safe haven at school, I will ensure one at home."

After much discussion, I insisted on a private tutor supplied by the school department. I could see his brain calculating the cost of such a request. That was not my concern. I left him to figure it out. Discussion was over.

I received a call informing me that my request was approved. The initial agreement was for three weeks of private tutoring. I was satisfied for the time being. Joshua was happy to feel safe, but very unhappy that poisons took precedence over his education.

Toxic Books

Staying home was very healthy for Joshua. The rash disappeared and his eyes stopped itching. His glands were back to normal and his energy level improved with each passing day.

Joshua realized he forgot one of his books at school that he needed for an assignment. He called the store. "Mom, can you pick it up for me today?" I jotted down his locker number and combination.

I left work to complete my assignment. When I delivered the book, he was studying in his room, "Here's the book you asked me to get for you, Josh." I left it on his nightstand and returned to work.

When I arrived home later in the day, he looked dizzy and confused. His glands were swollen and he was rubbing his eyes. "What happened?" I left a healthy child and came back to a sick one.

"I opened the book and reacted almost immediately," he replied. This was new to both of us. Had the chemicals permeated the whole school? Was everything contaminated with poisons? Joshua was now reacting to minute doses of the pesticide.

"Remember," I thought amongst my frustration, "there is always a solution to a problem. He had to have his school books. How could I make them safe?" I took the book outside into the fresh air and bright sunlight. I opened its pages and left it to air out for hours. The next day, he was able to use it with no reaction.

I share these stories with you to give you an understanding of how our bodies can become toxic and sensitive. Most of us go through life unconscious of possible exposures. Many learn to live with toxicity. This was not an option for Joshua. He understood clearly what was causing his reactions. He chose not to live with any of it. To do that, he had to make choices that ensured his ability to remain symptom free. The choices were not easy ones; but they were the right ones for him. He knew it did him no good to get angry, but he also knew he had a right to feel healthy in and out of school. What was a sixteen year old to do?

The End of a School Year

Joshua tried to return to school on May 26, almost five weeks from the day he left. As luck would have it, the school department spread wood chips around the outside of the building, as well as in the center courtyard. The problem was that there was a terrible odor being emitted from them. This odor encased the whole school. I was told there was no chemical added to these chips. The chemical was being produced as they aged. I'm not sure I believed it; but it did not matter. What mattered was that Joshua was sure it was not going to be good for him. He was excited to be back with his friends at school. Try as he might, he could not stay.

After two days, his glands were swelling and he was having problems breathing. His eyes itched and the rash reappeared under his arms. Enough again! He refused to go back to school. "I can't do it, Mom. As much as I want to be in school, I can't live like this."

The tutor was called back and he continued to be taught from home. He realized that besides his tutor and one of his teachers, no one else from the school really cared. I realized how unimportant one child is within the school community. Within a week, all Joshua's symptoms disappeared and he was healthy again. He liked the feeling of physical well being. He deserved no less. Joshua finished the school year at home, with high honors.

Joshua Needs Help Now

The members of the school board were about to feel my wrath. I decided it was time to recruit allies from the community.

My first thought was to type a letter explaining our struggle with the establishment. In it I shared Joshua's symptoms and his long history of missing school. I voiced my concerns over the possibility of how other children may be affected as well.

I mailed my letter to fifty of our customers and handed them out personally to every person who entered our store. I felt these were people who might share our concerns. After all, they frequented a health food store. I hoped a healthy environment was equally important. The letter asked parents to join me at the next school board meeting hoping to entice a few to speak on Joshua's behalf.

I realized that my best weapon would be Joshua himself. Until this time, I was doing all the guest appearances solo at the school board meetings. It was time I had a co-host and I wanted Joshua for the job. I approached him with my thoughts:

"Josh, I can't keep going to these meetings without you. My speech has become boring to them. They detach to the point of not even

listening any more. This is your fight. You have to join with me. I need you to speak at the next school board meeting."

His body language assured me that he was not happy with this request. He had his inferiority issues and they were apparent when confronted with those in authority. "I don't know if I can, Mom." I felt his fear, but there was no other option. I refused to take no for an answer.

As the day of the meeting approached, Joshua became more fearful. He had tons of excuses why he could not do it. None of them were legitimate. He finally gave me his best shot. "I'm afraid if I go near the school, I'll get sick again."

I tried to encourage him. "I understand your concerns. If the school does make you sick, it will be well worth it." Still he resisted. Finally, I put my foot down. "If you don't come to the meeting, I'm not going either. I'm in a losing battle without your support." He faced his fears and decided to join me.

The meeting proved to be a valuable experience. As the meeting convened, I nodded to Joshua. It was his time. "Just speak the truth." He slowly took his seat in front of the microphone. All eyes were on him. He unfolded the paper that contained his thoughts. His heart opened and without fear, he spoke face to face to those in authority.

By the time he finished, he possessed all the power in the room. I watched as each board member connected to his words. For a moment, they were one, feeling and experiencing somewhere deep inside themselves what Joshua was expressing. When he left that table, I knew change was about to happen. I did not know how, but I was sure we were not stuck any more.

One by one, people in the room followed Joshua's lead. His classmates supported his right to be in school. Parents who came to listen chose to voice their concerns for the safety of all children. A member of the Green Party arrived. He got wind of the meeting and presented information on the toxicity of the chemicals they were using at the school. The issue was no longer about Joshua. It was about an entire community demanding change.

The school board was so overwhelmed with speakers, they called a time out. "We get the point. We don't have to hear any more. We will take everyone's concerns into account."

A week later, we received a letter stating the school board had directed the staff to look into alternatives to chemicals. We were excited. Finally a breakthrough! We waited patiently for the next communication. None came. A month later, I called the superintendent's office and asked about the status of the school board's request. Again, there was no response.

I asked to keep us informed of any meetings or discussions that might take place regarding the fields. I heard nothing back. Joshua's initial excitement was turning back into frustration, "It's my senior year. I want to be in school."

If they continued to spray during the fall months, Joshua would not be able to get back to school until sometime late in November; and spring would be a repeat performance of the previous year. I refused to allow any more nonsense.

Who is Responsible for Joshua's Education?

July came and went and still, no response. We were impatient. Time was running out. Decisions had to be made before the end of August. Now what? I was running out of options, or was I? I started to think in a different direction. Joshua could not be in school. Joshua had a right to be in school. Who was responsible for him being in school? Who would help get him back into school? I made a list of people and places to call who might have an interest in his health and education:

-People with Disabilities
-The Department of Environmental Protection
-The CT State Department of Health
-The State Commissioner of Education

I contacted each one individually. I wasn't surprised at the replies; just disappointed.

People with Disabilities: *"His sensitivity was really not considered a disability. Sorry we can't help."*

The DEP: *"We encourage schools to use Integrative Pest Management Practices and alternatives to chemicals, but we don't have authority to enforce anything. Sorry, we can't help."*

CT State Department of Health: *"We understand how it could be a health concern, but it's really not our jurisdiction. Sorry, we can't help."*

The best one however, was the Commissioner of Education: *"It is not this office's responsibility to ensure Joshua is in school."*

My voice teetered on the edge of a scream. *"Okay, if it's not your responsibility, whose is it then?"*

I guess when one screams loud enough, someone responds eventually. My answer finally came from the Assistant Commissioner of Education. We talked extensively about Joshua's issue and after informing me there was nothing he could do, he did give me some valuable information.

"I think the office who might be able to help Joshua is the Office of Civil Rights in Massachusetts." *He offered me the number; I called immediately.*

The person on the other end listened. They asked questions. They transferred me to another number. Lo and behold, I was told they thought this might be a case they would consider. I promptly filed a complaint that Joshua was not being afforded his civil rights by being denied the right to receive an education at Killingly High School. We felt the school had an obligation to supply Joshua a healthy environment in order for him to get a proper education. After much deliberation, two lawyers from the office accepted Joshua's case. I felt relieved and satisfied.

Help Is Near

Having a lawyer from the Office of Civil Rights accept Joshua's case made a huge difference in how things were handled. Christine was my contact. When she called the superintendent's office, she received a quick response. I learned from this experience that life is a game. The trick is to learn the rules and then play to win. I learned the rules and I was playing to win.

It took time and a multitude of phone calls back and forth between Christine and the superintendent. After much deliberation Christine wanted to negotiate a settlement, so to speak.

"What do you feel is the greatest detriment to Joshua not being able to attend school?"

I knew the answer to that question, "I believe the weed killers have the greatest affect. They have the most severe warnings listed on the label and Joshua has experienced all the symptoms."

I conferred with Joshua. "Do you think if the school stopped spraying weed killers you might be able to attend school without getting sick?" Neither of us could be certain, but we were willing to try.

With OCR's intervention, a compromise between the parties was reached:

The school department would discontinue the practice of spraying weed killers on the high school fields and Joshua would have final say if the school were a healthy environment for him.

I also felt that his symptoms improved dramatically after a rainfall, which made me realize that the chemicals were most likely being washed away. Although that was a concern for me, I kept my focus on Joshua's health. I renegotiated the agreement to include another section:

The fields would be watered immediately after application of any chemical.

Much to my satisfaction, the school board agreed. There were no weed killers applied in September of Joshua's senior year, and the fields were promptly watered after the application of the chemical fertilizers. Joshua did not lose a single day of school. He was happy and his report card showed straight A's for the quarter.

He is gifted and talented when he is healthy and happy, and he was very happy to be back at school with his friends. We walk the path of high school only once in life, and we should not miss a single minute of it. Joshua had already missed way too much.

It took years, but we accomplished what we set out to do which was to provide a safe environment for everyone in our school and on our fields. Joshua was the instrument for that change. He's never regretted what he had to do.

Joshua the Teacher

Our mission to change what we sprayed on the fields at Killingly High School became widely known throughout the town. Before long parents were recognizing that their children were experiencing the same symptoms as Joshua. The store became a haven for healthy discussions regarding how to help their children heal. If a child accompanied their parent and Joshua was available, I would ask him to speak directly to these children. Joshua assured them that it's okay to be different and being healthy is a right no one should be denied.

The children Joshua spoke to left with an understanding that they were not really so different after all. The only difference between them and others was the awareness of what made them ill. By sharing our problems and solutions, we continued to work toward a healthier environment for everyone. Together, Joshua and I learned that we can change the way the world heals, one person at a time.

Chapter Eight

~ The Auditory Learner ~

Joshua was very different from other children because he was aware of what made him ill and he took responsibility to fix himself. When he was healthy, he could focus in school. When he was not healthy, his school work suffered. Sometimes it was difficult to separate his chemical sensitivities with his reading disability. Were they the same?

When Joshua entered second grade, he had little interest in reading, and the little reading he managed to accomplish was at a snail's pace. There were times he downright refused to read at all; he found it too frustrating. His reading level was below what was "expected" of him at this age. However, I began to notice that although he was a slow reader, he had no problem comprehending the material. It was as though he did not like reading, but enjoyed learning. I was confused. What really is the issue?

One day Joshua came home with a note that stated he was being offered an opportunity to enroll in a remedial reading program. The school felt he was not reading to potential and wanted to give him extra help so he could improve his reading skills.

Joshua was devastated. He felt stupid and foolish. He came home that day distraught. "Josh, you are not stupid. You are very smart. You are just having a difficult time reading. Maybe the remedial reading program will help you read better. Reading is important. Why not try to see if it helps?"

With my coaxing, he agreed to attend the program. Each week he was called to his special classroom where he received special attention in reading. What bothered him most was being singled out of the classroom in the middle of the day. All eyes were on him. His peers knew that he was in a special class for those who could not do something well. He felt belittled and inferior. I felt sad that he was made to feel different again, and yet, I wanted to make sure he had every opportunity to learn to read to his fullest potential.

I encouraged his reading by taking him to the library often. His interests were varied. This one particular day he chose a large book on dinosaurs. Dinosaurs and animals were two of his favorite topics. It was not a book that would seem appropriate for a second grader to read; but I did not want to dictate his choices nor did I want to discourage his reading. We checked the book out and took it home.

That evening he brought me his new library book and asked me to read to him. He loved being read to even if he did not like reading himself. As I read this complicated material, I had to wonder how much he understood. I felt some of it was too complicated for me, never mind a second grader! "Josh, do you know what I just read to you?"

His answer was simple, "Yes." He then proceeded to reiterate back to me, word for word the entire previous paragraph.

It was in that moment I realized Joshua was an auditory learner. He learned best while listening. As he was being read to, he was memorizing the words in his head. I then started to pay attention to his reading skills. He had a need to memorize every word. It made his reading extremely slow. It wasn't that he could not read; he just read differently. There was more to learn from my auditory learner:

On a separate trip to the library, Joshua found the book, "Bo Knows Bo," an autobiography about the baseball player Bo Jackson. Again, I did not think this book was appropriate for a second grader, especially one who had a hard time reading. Joshua thought otherwise. He was excited to find this book. "This is a great book. I can't wait to

106

start reading it when I get home!" Why would I deny him such excitement?

Each evening Joshua made his way up to his room so he could be alone with Bo Jackson. As I watched him slowly move through Bo's book I wondered out loud, "Josh, if you can read this book, why can't you read the books at school?"

His reply was simple and profound as always, "Mom, the books they make us read at school are stupid books! I don't want to read them." Joshua was consciously choosing not to read books he had no interest in. Why didn't the teachers know this?

I learned from Joshua by taking the time to find out what was really going on with his so-called problems. His major problems were the way he was being taught and the books he was required to read. Soon thereafter Joshua "graduated" from remedial reading. The book, *Bo Knows Bo,* was the inspiration for his graduation. The school had no idea.

The school really was not interested in how Joshua learned differently. To them, all children were the same and they had to learn the same way. Otherwise, they were deemed failures. The school's agenda did not meet Joshua's needs. That was not acceptable. My job was to ensure that Joshua's needs were met at school and at home.

I started to research learning techniques. There were many studies conducted about the different ways children learn. Three of the most common are:

Visual-- I must see it to believe it (faith based)

Auditory--I must hear it to understand it (analytically based)

Kinetic--I must touch it to create it (building based)

There are children who learn by all three methods; and there are children who don't. It does not make one child better than another; just different. I was fascinated.

The studies proved that children learn differently, yet schools continued to teach all children the same. I consulted our superintendent of schools.

"I have been doing research about learning methods and I am learning that Joshua is an auditory learner. He learns by hearing. Are you familiar with these studies?"

"Yes, I have read about them," was his noncommittal reply.

"Then why are we teaching children the same way? Why not use this information to help children become successful by all the means available?" He had no answer to my question, and his body language assured me that learning techniques were not going to change soon.

Obviously, I could not wait for the educated to catch up to the research. Recognizing Joshua's auditory abilities would help him become successful throughout his life. It made sense to me that Joshua needed an auditory teacher to meet his auditory needs. Each summer, I went to the guidance office and explained Joshua's learning skills. I then asked the same question, "Who are the teachers who enjoy lecturing in the classroom?"

Joshua may have been a slow reader; he did not have to suffer because of it. With the right tools and teachers, Joshua learned how to use his auditory skills to his advantage. The guidance counselors were happy to help with Joshua's needs. So were his teachers. Joshua continued to do well in school because he and I were involved in the decisions that ensured his success.

High school was more of a challenge. By his junior year he came home with a required reading list that was way too long for his liking.

"Mom, I'm expected to read all these books during the year. How will I ever get it all done?" After a little deliberation, I came up with a solution that I knew would work well for Joshua. I also knew the school system would not approve. I decided not to share it with them.

"Josh, all the books you have to read are on tapes. Tomorrow I will take you to the library and you can see what is available." He smiled at me with that beautiful smile that said it all. He thought that was a great idea.

Book reports and books on tape were interconnected in the same way listening and learning were now interconnected. He loved listening to books on tape which in turn helped him love learning. Joshua was now a successful reader, an auditory reader, but a reader nonetheless.

It was important for Joshua to come to peace with his special way of learning. As he mastered his way of healing he also mastered his way of learning. We allowed him that right and privilege. Success is not based on being the same as everyone else; it is based on honoring our differences. Joshua graduated with high honors.

Note from Joshua: Upon reading this chapter, Joshua was quick to point out that it was in second grade that he was poisoned by the water at school. His inability to focus, concentrate and read during that time was greatly affected, and it took more than a month before the cause of the problem was recognized. Hence, he was labeled remedial. The truth was and still is that Joshua will always be a slow reader; it does not make him a bad reader. His abilities to retain vast amounts of information and his auditory capabilities have proven to be a huge advantage as he moves through life.

Chapter Nine

~ Magical Sensitive Child ~

I was not sure where to place this chapter, but I was sure it was important to share. Before being influenced by the thoughts and beliefs of others, Joshua believed in himself and the magic that surrounded him. Magical gifts are a part of every sensitive being. To connect to these magical powers, the mind and body must be free of chemicals and toxins. This pure state opens channels that connect to one's divine nature. Joshua was very connected.

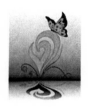

I loved Joshua's magical gifts. I encouraged each one from the moment he shared them with me. Had I thought to discredit his powers and had I tried to convince him that magic was not real, his gifts would have been lost and forgotten over time. Instead he allowed himself to be open to the many possibilities life had to offer.

Let the Sun Shine!

When Joshua was five years old, he learned that he could speak to the clouds. One day, he shared his secret with me.

"I can make the rain go away. All I have to do is speak to the clouds and the sun will come out." He stood there waiting for me to discredit him, to tell him speaking to the clouds was not possible. It never occurred to me to do such a thing.

I felt honored that Joshua wanted to share his secret with me. I believed in him and I believed he had special gifts. The smile on my face assured him I did not think him weird. I thought him special and I was grateful that he believed in himself. To his secret I replied, "I think you are very lucky to have such special gifts." That was all he needed. He was looking for assurance that magic was real. He walked away feeling confident and secure in himself.

If he had been in another home, the door may have been shut on his gift that day. If I said to him, "That's silly, no one can do that," I may have denied myself opportunities to see how powerful he was, and I would not be sharing these magical stories with you today. Because I chose otherwise, Joshua continued to speak to the clouds and the rain.

His beliefs were strong and his abilities intensified over time. On many a rainy day, Joshua went outside and talked to the clouds. Before long, the clouds moved quickly across the sky and the sun soon appeared. When adverse weather was predicted for a family event, Joshua went to work ensuring a sunny day. Although these events could be perceived as coincidences, there was one particular day that could not be denied.

It was the weekend of Halloween and we were hosting a "Haunted Trail" in the woods behind our home. When we awoke that morning, the sky opened up and released buckets of rain. The rain was so heavy that within a few moments of being outside, you were soaked from head to toe. The morning weather forecast gave us little hope, as this dismal day was predicted to continue into the night. Our haunted trail was scheduled to begin at four o'clock, just as the day turned to dusk. At noon, I decided to ask Joshua for help.

"Joshua, I know you can talk to the rain. I have seen you do it many times. Do you think you could get the sun to come out for our haunted trail?"

Joshua never fledged at the opportunity to use his magical powers for the good of the many. He quickly answered, "Okay, mom," and walked out the door that led him to the back field. I watched him and although I don't know the words he used, his eyes were intense. I could almost see the energy being emitted from his little body. When he came back inside, he was drenched. He explained, "I talked to the clouds and the rain. I hope they heard me."

Still the rain continued. At two o'clock in the afternoon, I said, "Josh, maybe they didn't hear you. Can you try again?"

Joshua again went out into the fields. His determination showed through the expression on his face. His head was tilted toward the sky, his eyes blinking with each raindrop that fell, his lips moving as if in prayer. Again, Joshua came back inside certain that he had been heard by the angels of the rain and the angels of the clouds, but the rain continued to drench the fields almost to the point of flooding. "I don't understand what's wrong," Joshua said. "I did everything I know how to do, but it isn't working."

I sat down with Joshua and explained, "Sometimes, things don't turn out like we want them to. Sometimes the angels have different plans. I do appreciate that you made the effort." He seemed comforted by the words, so I continued, "I know how hard you tried. Maybe it was just supposed to rain today and sometimes we have to accept that the angels know what's best."

Soon after making peace with the angels' decision, a strange thing happened. Joshua and I were sitting together under the safety of our covered porch putting the final touches together for our haunted trail. Halloween must go on! The rain continued to pour down around us until exactly at four o'clock, the rain stopped. It was a quick stop as though someone suddenly turned off the faucets. Then as quickly as the rain stopped, the sun broke through the clouds and poured its warming, drying rays upon the rain soaked fields. It was a magical moment for Joshua and me.

We looked at each other and laughed because we knew. We knew that the angels of the clouds and the angels of the rain heard Joshua as he spoke throughout the day. They understood that the sun was only needed at four o'clock in the afternoon. I thanked the sun for joining us. Slowly it disappeared behind the trees in the far corner of our yard. Our haunted trail took place on a beautiful, clear and starry evening.

Bird Talk

Joshua had other gifts. As well as speaking to the clouds, he also spoke to the living creatures of the Earth. It was a popular pastime for Joshua. Occasionally I got a glimpse of this magical sight.

When he first started school, his sister and the other neighborhood children were older. His bus came a little later, and each morning he waited at the bus stop by himself. I kept an eye on him from my upstairs bedroom window. Joshua was not aware that I spent my mornings at that window. Many times I saw a side of him no one else was allowed to witness. There was one particular morning when he was in the second grade.

Spring was in the air, the trees were in full bloom and the day was bright and clear. Joshua was alone in the yard waiting for his bus to arrive. Joshua did not mind being alone. He always found ways to occupy his time and his thoughts. At that moment, I was thinking it would be nice if he had a friend to wait with him; however, Joshua had other ideas.

Within minutes, I watched as he called a flock of birds to his feet. One by one, they flew directly in front of him. It seemed as though they were patiently waiting for something to happen. I wondered if they were looking for food, however, he had no food for them. This was not about eating. This was about talking and listening. It was about company. The birds stayed at his feet as he spoke to them until the bus arrived. Then they quickly dispersed and Joshua went off to school.

I never bothered to ask what he talked to them about. It did not matter to me. I felt blessed to have the opportunity to watch his gifts and allow his magic to evolve without interference.

A Prison Made of Glass

Another fond memory of Joshua and nature was the day he caught a beautiful yellow butterfly in a jar. It was a perfect summer day. The air was warm and the wild flowers and grasses filled the field outside our home. The whole neighborhood was out enjoying the summer air.

Joshua could not believe he caught a butterfly in a jar. His eyes were wide with excitement! He held the jar upside down on top of the palm of his hand. He ran from neighbor to neighbor showing off his new "pet" butterfly.

"Look at my beautiful butterfly," he said with a huge grin of accomplishment. Everyone was quite impressed except the poor petrified butterfly. She was flapping her wings as fast as she could, trying to make her escape back to freedom. It did not take her long to realize she was trapped in a prison made of glass.

Through the jar, I felt the horror she was experiencing. When Joshua finally got to me, his face was beaming with pride as he showed me his rare catch. "Isn't she beautiful?" he exclaimed.

I had to admit she was beautiful. I knew that Joshua was not seeing the truth at that moment. He was only seeing what he wanted to see. He believed that he owned this butterfly. He held the fate of her future in the palm of his hand. That was a powerful feeling to experience.

It was not my job to tell Joshua how to handle any situation. It was my job to guide and teach him. So I redirected his thoughts to what was really happening through his glass jar at that moment. "Joshua, look at the butterfly through the jar. What do you see?"

He stopped for a long moment and stared into the jar. For the first time, he did not see her as his butterfly, but as a frightened living being trapped in a cage. His dark brown eyes turned from joy to concern and then to compassion. I watched as he felt the same intensity his butterfly was experiencing through his very soul. His emotions changed instantly from feelings of excitement to feelings of despair. He could see and feel the same fear his butterfly was experiencing. He knew he had to send her home. Joshua shared her beauty with all of us. She had nothing else to offer.

For a few rare moments, he held onto her jar. His love and compassion for this tiny insect was clearly being emitted through his eyes and heart. "I need to let her go, don't I?" Then he joyously removed the jar off his hand to free his beautiful friend.

I expected that butterfly to move herself quickly away from her glass prison, but to my surprise, she sat directly on top of his hand and stared him straight in the eye. I heard no voice, but I have no doubt that the yellow butterfly knew exactly what she was doing. She realized she was being granted her freedom, and she stopped for a few moments to say, "Thank you my friend," and through Joshua's eyes, I could hear him say, "You're welcome." Only then did she fly back home to safety.

Denying Himself

Joshua's ability to speak to the animals, the birds, the insects, and the clouds continued for a few more years. With any gift, the power comes from the belief inside. One rainy day, I asked Joshua if he would speak to the clouds for me. On that sad day he turned to me with anger in his voice, "That's dumb. No one can do that." He no longer embraced his magic, but transformed it into fear. Peer pressure had taken over and he refused to be special any longer. He just wanted to fit in.

My heart was broken that day, but I knew this was his journey, not mine. Just as I supported him when he accepted his gifts, I also had to support him when he denied them. He had to follow his own path.

I knew his magic was hidden, but not forgotten. I understood he needed space to see who he was and who he wanted to be. I also knew in my heart that one day the memory of his mission would return. I had no doubt that his mission was an important one. So important that God ensured that no chemical would interfere with what he needed to do.

I said a prayer that morning for the future. I prayed that when Joshua eventually worked through his peer pressure, he would come back to embrace the magic he was born with. Inside, however, I knew that everything was perfect just the way it was. I would wait for the day when he would accept his powers again.

Chapter Ten

~ Alternative Medicines ~

Allopathic medicines were never an option where Joshua was concerned. I quickly realized that chemicals were the problem and drugs were chemicals. I had to look for alternative ways to help my son heal. As the store grew, so did my knowledge of holistic healing modalities. I studied many therapies and introduced into Joshua's world those that I felt complemented his healing. I began with homeopathy.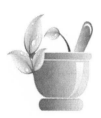

I was attracted to homeopathic remedies from the moment I explored alternative healing practices. Homeopathy "felt" right to me. However, there was only one homeopathic doctor nearby and he was not taking new patients. I had to study on my own.

I purchased self help homeopathic books and a homeopathic kit that contained the most common remedies for home situations. I attended seminars and classes that offered anything that remotely resembled any type of alternative therapy. I was especially drawn to lectures on the topic of vibration medicines. With all this information now firmly planted in my mind, I was not surprised when I was required to put my knowledge to the test:

We lived on a long winding country road. Across the street was a field which was home to a number of horses who spent their time grazing on the grass. Joshua was not quite two years old when my friend and neighbor asked if she could take him for a walk to visit the horses. Within ten minutes, Kathy was rushing back to the house with Joshua in her arms. She was frantic.

"I don't know what happened. When we got close to the horses, his eyes began to water and he started to sneeze. Now look at him!"

I barely recognized my son as he peered out at me through two slits sitting on top of what appeared to be golf balls placed in the sockets where his eyes used to be. Of course, I knew these were Joshua's eyes, but I did not know why they were so swollen. It appeared he could still see me through these two little slits that now encased his eyes. I wondered for how long?

I was scared. I didn't know what to do. For the first time I thought about rushing him to the nearest hospital. That thought was soon interrupted by another, "What would a hospital have to offer him? With his history, chemicals were out of the question; and if they insisted, would allopathic therapies trigger more reactions?"

I recently purchased a book called "Everybody's Guide to Homeopathic Remedies." I ran to get my copy and looked up eye problems. I read that the homeopathic remedy called "Apis" might work for eyes that looked swollen as if they were filled with fluid. I looked back at Josh. His eyes could be mistaken for two little balloons filled with water.

"I'm going to get my homeopathic kit. Stay with Josh! I want to see if I have this remedy called Apis." I opened the box only once when I first received it; it had not been opened since. I wasn't even sure what remedies it contained.

The thirty-two vials were arranged in alphabetical order; Apis was one of them. I held the vial in my hand and thought about the possible consequences. "What if I give this to him and he gets worse?" Kathy had no response. She waited as I made my decision. Joshua watched through his two small slits trusting I would know how to help him. I felt even more fearful.

Finally, I pushed my fears aside and popped a few pellets on Joshua's tongue. Ever so slowly, Kathy and I witnessed what might be called a miracle. With each passing moment, Joshua's eyes slowly turned back to his normal state. In two minutes there was no indication they were ever swollen.

Kathy and I looked at each other. We knew our lives were altered. Could healing be so quick, easy and noninvasive? In that moment, I became an advocate of homeopathic medicines.

A Homeopathic Physician

Joshua's original pediatrician had always been patient with me and I appreciated him. He listened to my lengthy explanations about chemical sensitivities and the merits of organic ingredients. I'm not sure he was completely convinced of my arguments. There were times he must have thought I was downright crazy. To him, Joshua probably seemed like a semi-normal kid who was asthmatic, a bit temperamental, and on the fast track to receiving heavy doses of Ritalin.

Of course, I was seeing things quite differently. Fortunately, he and I had one very important thing in common. He was not the type of doctor who pushed drugs onto children, and I was not the type of mother who approved of their use. I was focused on finding real solutions to Joshua's problems.

About a year after the Apis incident, I heard that the local homeopathic doctor was accepting new patients. This was a rare occurrence, as his services were in high demand and he was limited by the number of patients he could effectively treat. I felt an urgency to become a patient of homeopathy.

I called Joshua's pediatrician and explained the situation. He was quite aware that holistic therapy was the course I wanted to explore with my children. He knew that alternative medicines would become a way of life for me, and he had doubts he could meet my future needs and accept my strange beliefs. He gave me his blessing, and I scheduled Joshua's first visit with his new homeopathic doctor.

The experience of a first homeopathic visit is different from anything I experienced with any other doctor. You don't take your clothes off. It feels more like a conference, sharing as much information as possible about the patient, physically and emotionally. Dr. Bill was genuinely interested in Joshua's thoughts and feelings and took time to listen. Joshua sat at my feet playing with the few toys I took with me to keep him entertained. I probed my memory to share as much information with Dr. Bill as I could remember.

We spent an hour and a half going over Joshua's extensive history of allergies and reactions. We talked about his temper tantrums and rashes. We talked about his breathing and mucus problems. We talked about everything I could think of and still Dr. Bill would say, "What else?"

I explained everything I learned about chemicals in the environment and chemicals in the food and how he reacted differently to different situations. Again, Dr. Bill would say, "What else?" Finally I had to ask, "Isn't that enough?" Dr. Bill laughed. He took the information he gathered from our visit and began plugging it into his computer.

I learned that day that there can be no secrets to get the desired results from a remedy. Everything must be placed on the table. The truth is imperative to heal. We cannot hide our issues nor can we pretend they don't exist. The more information a homeopathic doctor has at his disposal, the better the chances for finding the correct constitutional remedy up front.

After a few minutes of research, Dr. Bill finally prescribed for Joshua the remedy called Staphysagria.

Joshua's Constitutional Remedy

A constitutional remedy is one that addresses the symptoms of the whole person. It is based on the principle of "like cures like." For instance, the situation with Apis worked so well because Apis is made from bee venom. If stung by a bee, swelling, itching, or irritation of the area might occur. The same was true with Joshua's eyes, they were swollen, itchy and irritated. Thereby, this remedy would be useful to help cure the same symptoms as if a bee had been the culprit.

Homeopathy is a medicine that heals through the vibration of the body. It helps to heal physical symptoms because it is helping the body balance itself emotionally and mentally. With homeopathy, either it works or it doesn't. If it doesn't work, you try another remedy until you find the correct one; the one the body responds to.

There are no side effects per se. What one might experience is called "a proving," which means the body may respond to the remedy by either a physical or emotional response. A proving is a positive sign that the remedy has touched on something. It allows the body to boost its immune system to begin the healing process. It does not hide symptoms; instead it assists the body in healing symptoms.

The purpose of working with Joshua's constitutional remedy was to help his body become less sensitive over time. I had not heard of Staphysagria until Dr. Bill prescribed it. It was clear to me why Dr. Bill chose this remedy for Joshua.

According to The Homeopathy Bible by Ambika Wauters, "The Staphysagria patient is very sensitive and has violent and passionate outbursts...It is useful for illnesses that have been caused by a person bottling up their anger inside. They... are sensitive to sounds, sights, taste and touch..."

Joshua received his first dose of Staphysagria that day, and we scheduled a two-week follow up. Two weeks later, I felt I had seen a difference in his reactions. It's hard to remember now exactly what pinpointed my feelings, but I remember thinking something was different about him. Something appeared better about his overall attitude. After listening to the stories surrounding the previous two weeks, Dr. Bill also felt we were on the right track. Joshua received another dose.

I saw improvement gradually occur. Each new dose seemed to have a longer lasting affect. Our visits soon turned into every other month, and eventually every six months. I learned when Joshua might need an additional dose of his remedy by paying attention to his reactions and attitude. I also learned that whenever Joshua was affected by a chemical, the sooner I gave him a dose of his remedy, the less severe the reaction. I learned to keep a vial of Staphysagria with us wherever we went.

I felt fortunate to have been introduced to alternative healing modalities. Joshua had many tools at his disposal to help him heal. Drugs were never one of them. Instead, along with organic food and natural cleaning products, homeopathic medicines found their way into Joshua's medicine cabinet.

To Immunize or Not to Immunize

With Joshua's long history of sensitivities, injecting his body with foreign substances did not feel good, so I avoided giving Joshua very many immunizations. Of the few I allowed, he had already had one noted reaction. I was not comfortable taking chances on another injection that could prove detrimental.

I voiced my concerns to Dr. Bill. We talked a lot about it, round and round we went. Finally, I asked him directly, "If he were your son, what would you do?" He offered me his honest opinion with the understanding that I had to make my own choices for my child. I honored his thoughts and beliefs and was grateful that he was willing to share them with me.

I began to give serious thought regarding my choices for Joshua. I knew in my heart that injecting foreign substances into his sensitive body may have serious consequences. I began researching the issue extensively and noted the growing concerns attached to immunizations and autistic behaviors. What if Joshua's sensitive nature made him a candidate for such a reaction? I chose to take no chances. I consciously chose to stop any further injections.

That is a choice I did not take lightly, but I made it without fear. I trusted the choices I made to create a healthy environment; I also had to trust my decisions concerning immunizations. Outside, in the real world, I knew I would be challenged, especially when it was time to face the school system.

School systems have certain requirements, one of which is a long list of immunizations. Joshua's list was way too short for their liking. I had to be educated to stand up to those in power. My choices were tied to enhancing Joshua's immune system with natural means. How would I get the schools to accept my beliefs? I would find out soon enough when it was time for Joshua to enter the public school system.

Joshua was getting ready for his first day of kindergarten. He was excited and ready to leave his nest. I was concerned. There were the issues of snacks and drinks, and chemicals in his new environment. However, these issues seemed small compared to what I would have to face. Joshua simply did not meet their immunization requirements.

I was told by a number of our customers at the store that there was no need to worry. All you have to do is fill out a religious waiver form. "Does a priest have to sign it?" I asked. It had been many years since I belonged to any organized religion.

I soon learned, "The only one who has to sign the form is you." That sounded way too easy. With as much courage as I could muster, I made an appointment to see the school nurse a few days before school started.

"I would like to fill out a religious waver form for Joshua's immunizations." She was a bit taken aback by my request. It became obvious that very few parents ventured from the norm and asked for the "secret form." I was one of those parents.

"I do remember such a form. Rarely has anyone ever asked for it," she politely explained. I watched as she tried to remember where she may have filed these unused forms. She began digging into the bottom of her filing cabinet, searching for a form that was filed where no one might be able to find it. Eventually she stood up with form in hand.

"Ah, here it is," she proclaimed proudly.

My request for that form did not seem to affect her one way or another. She was simply doing her duty and I was doing mine. She handed me the form and stepped aside. I filled it out and signed my name.

This ceremony occurred each time Joshua entered a new school: middle school, high school and college. The middle school nurse thought me a terrible parent; the high school nurse thought I was empowered and the college nurse, well she was our greatest challenge.

When it was time to enter college, Joshua was old enough to make his own decisions. When his college forms arrived, there were two requirements Joshua had issues with. One was the long list of immunizations deemed necessary; the other was mandatory health insurance that he felt he would never use. It was now his responsibility to deal with these situations; I felt he was prepared.

"Mom, can you come with me to talk to the school about these forms?" I was happy to accompany him. I had been through it so many times, I was becoming a professional.

It took a while to find the nurse's office on campus. It was impressive with dark polished wooden doors and walls, a bit overwhelming in stature. I pushed open the doors and stood at the desk waiting for the receptionist to recognize our presence. Once we had her attention, I got right to the point. "I would like to sign a religious waiver for Joshua's required immunizations," I explained.

The receptionist immediately went into defense mode and I watched as the hair on the back of her neck stood upright. My protective shields were ready and I was able to avoid the energetic darts she emitted toward the two of us. "Are you sure about that? If there is an outbreak of measles on campus, Joshua will have to leave the school grounds for at least two weeks!"

That did not seem unreasonable to either of us. He already missed three months in high school. Two weeks sounded like a short vacation. "That's fine," I answered back.

She immediately became indignant. How dare I think missing two weeks of school would be fine? She threw the paper at us and informed me that Joshua was required to fill out the form as an adult. Joshua took on his adult duty and signed the waiver.

As he handed the waiver back to her, I voiced my next request. "We also want to refuse the health insurance coverage. Is there a form for that as well?" That put her over the edge. She left the office and returned with reinforcements. Her supervisor marched in ready to take on the new recruit that dared to usurp her authority.

"I understand you are refusing Joshua's health insurance?"

"Yes," I answered. "With Joshua's extensive health history and allergies, I am concerned what a doctor or hospital might try to put into his body. It's best if his health insurance were left up to us to make a decision based on individual circumstances."

She dared counter me. "Joshua is eighteen now. He is responsible for his health insurance and his own decisions."

"That's fine." I turned my focus toward Joshua. "Josh, do you want to sign a waiver for health insurance?"

Joshua looked at the supervisor and with certainty he replied, "Yes, I want to sign the waiver. If I'm responsible for health insurance, I can assure you I have no money to pay for it anyway."

Anger permeated the room. Who were these people who defied our rules and regulations? She shot back with her best effort, "What if you get leukemia?" she demanded. Joshua had no idea how to answer that question. I moved him aside.

As calmly as I could, I replied, "Why would you want my son to get leukemia?"

She was thrown off course. "I don't want him to get leukemia," she assured me.

"Then why would you say such a thing? We believe that what we speak is what we create in life, and leukemia is not one of the things we are trying to create. I would appreciate it if you would respect our beliefs."

Possibly for the first time in her life, the "general" was speechless. She quickly turned around and retreated back into her office. Joshua signed the waiver and we left feeling at peace with our decisions.

We hoped we taught the office staff a valuable lesson that day. Although our beliefs were extremely different, it did not make one right or wrong. It made them different. All we desired was to be honored for our differences.

The supervisor tried desperately to pass her fears onto us. We did not want them nor would we accept them. We left her fears back at the office with her and her staff. Joshua had another moment of empowerment. He was learning how to stand strong in his own beliefs, not having to take on the beliefs that others may try to force upon him. These were all very powerful lessons.

In his sophomore year, Joshua decided he wanted to transfer from Bryant College in Rhode Island to the University of Colorado in Boulder. Of course, proof of immunizations was requested for the transfer. It is amazing how the same situation can turn out so differently:

I called the medical office to request a religious waiver. The gentleman who answered asked, "What is a religious waiver? I've never heard of it."

I explained as best I could. "If a person does not choose to be immunized, there is a religious waiver form that can be signed to excuse them from the college policies."

He replied, "That's interesting. I don't know anything about it. Why don't you just type up a letter and I'll put it in his file?"

A simple procedure for a simple request! There was no argument or discussion. In his mind as in my own, I was allowed my differences.

Joshua's Homeopathic Medicine Cabinet

There are hundreds, and maybe thousands, of different homeopathic remedies. It was not necessary for me to learn all of them. As time went on, I began to see a pattern developing. Different poisons created different reactions; which in turn, different reactions called for different medicines. I was blessed to have the advantage of kinesiology or muscle testing at my finger tips. It was a valuable tool in helping me determine what Joshua needed to counter one of his reactive moments.

Each child is unique and different. A remedy that was good for Joshua may not be the correct remedy for another child. A homeopathic doctor can help determine the correct constitutional remedy based on history including reactions and symptoms.

It was very important for me and Joshua to feel safe and comfortable with our physician of choice. Dr. Bill did not always have to agree with me; however, he did have to respect my choices. I had the final say in what was best for my child. Dr. Bill and I got on well together.

Over time, Joshua's medicine cabinet was filled with the remedies he used the most. We kept each on hand for emergencies. Joshua responded well to these medicines. He took them without fear of any chemical reaction. The best part about homeopathy is they do not spoil with age. They are as effective today as they were years ago.

— Arnica Montana is used to treat trauma, shock or injury. Joshua was an outdoorsy kind of kid. He also loved to play sports and Arnica was often needed to help his body heal from the trauma of injuries. I kept a vial in the glove box just in case. I once heard a story of how Arnica became known as a healing plant.

The farmers of long ago watched the mountain goats high on top of the hillsides of their village. Whenever a goat fell and was injured, the goat immediately grazed on the arnica plant. The farmers noticed that the goats healed quickly from the injuries and trauma.

— Apis was used during times of swelling for both of his eyes and throat and always if he were stung by a bee or wasp.

— Cantharis Vescatoria was kept for times of bladder and kidney irritation, of which Joshua experienced during his healing process. Cantharis helped move the irritation through quickly.

- Euphrasia is specific to helping symptoms of the eyes and mucus membranes. Itching, tearing, and pain of the eyes are common when Euphrasia is called for and we used it often for Joshua's allergic reactions, especially when he was close to horses.

- Hypericum is used for injuries to the nerves and nerve endings. This along with Arnica is helpful to carry in one's trauma kit. Catching a finger in the car door is the perfect moment for Hypericum to do its job.

- Magnesia Phosphorica is used to nourish the muscular system. It can be helpful for pains associated with muscular tension including cramps, headaches and muscle aches. Joshua used this tissue salt during times when his sensitive digestive system did not absorb magnesium well.

- Natrum Phosphoricum is the acid balancer of the body. A dose of Nat Phos will often help relieve the symptoms of heartburn. Fears create an acidic state in the body and Joshua was often full of fear. Nat Phos helped balance his system.

- Silica is the main constituent of the hair, skin and nails. It also helps the body cleanse and eliminate matter that should have been discharged but got stuck in the body, such as sties, boils, or cysts. High school was a time Silica was needed.

- Staphysagria was and continues to be Joshua's constitutional remedy. It is for sensitive people who may have violent angry outbursts. These people also have acute senses of taste and smell. This remedy spelled Joshua!

- Symphytum is the bone knitter. It is given to clients who have broken or fractured bones, but only after the bone has been set in the proper place. This was a very important remedy when Joshua broke his collar bone.

The Herbal Cleansers

To heal, Joshua needed medicines that helped his body cleanse and strengthen his digestive organs and glands. Chemicals would clog his liver and spleen. During his high school years, the toxicity levels were deep into his lymphatic system. I learned as much as I could about how herbal cleansers worked. It was imperative that we kept the flow of toxins through the normal channels of his body. Herbal cleansers found a place among Joshua's homeopathic remedies.

When he was younger, Dandelion Root was my first choice. It is a gentle tonic that I felt safe using even when he was quite little. As he got older, we used the appropriate cleansers dependent upon the toxicity and the symptoms created. Muscle testing helped determine our choices.

– Dandelion Root is a gentle tonic that I used from the time Joshua was very little. It can help remove toxins from the liver, spleen and gall bladder; it can also help flush the bladder and kidneys. He still uses this herb today.

– Burdock Root is a blood and lymphatic cleanser and was introduced during the years when cysts became a symptom of chemical poisoning.

– Yellowdock is a deep acting blood cleanser and helped with skin rashes and lymphatic drainage through the spleen.

– Milk Thistle helped to protect and strengthen his liver from the onslaught of chemicals.

My ability to understand and use these types of medicines were a gift that enabled Joshua to heal and for me to learn. Our lives have been blessed with everything we need to be healthy.

There Is Always More to Learn

I was thrilled to be learning so much through Joshua. He had clearly shown me the importance of organic food and pure water. He enforced my belief that a clean environment ensured his health and safety. He was now teaching me about detoxifying chemicals through the organs that help with this process: *the liver, spleen mucus membranes and lymphatic system.*

Along with everything else, homeopathic remedies were becoming our medicine of choice to help him move energy that became stuck in his system. I enjoyed Joshua's school of higher education.

However, I began to realize that there was more to healing than just working the physical body. What it was eluded me at that moment. Time would soon reveal the lesson he was destined to teach next. I waited patiently for his next indicator.

I was certain, however, that my earlier thoughts of the person Joshua came to be were true. He was on a divine mission to teach through his own personal healing experiences. What he was about to teach me would again change the course of my life and the lives of many others that were willing to learn: *our emotions create our physical symptoms.*

Chapter Eleven

~ Healing Through Emotions ~

Flower essences came into our world at just the appropriate moment, and healing took on a new and exciting reality. Flower essences, along with muscle testing, kept us focused on health.

It was 1987. We had been in business for five years and opened our second health food store. We were busy with the two stores and our children that now totaled three. Money was tight; we invested it on a clean environment and organic food. We enjoyed the life we were creating.

Like Joshua, I loved learning and attended as many seminars on alternative healing as we could afford. One day Ken was reading from one of his order books, "Hey Lin, Cornucopia is offering to pay for level I of a seminar offered by the Bach Institute. Each store is allowed to send one person for free. Is that something that interests you?" I liked the word "free."

I was familiar with the Bach flower essences; however, I had minimal understanding of their uses. With a little research I learned they were used to help heal the emotional body. That sparked my interest. "I think I will take advantage of Cornucopia's offer."

This was another life altering decision. The guinea pigs of my past (my friends and family) offered to participate in this new healing experiment. What we experienced together was magical. With the use of flower essences, we were recognizing our patterns of behavior and becoming accountable for our choices.

Seeing Through the Eyes of Truth

In August of 2000, I completed the three levels necessary to be deemed a Bach Flower Practitioner. By that time, I was using the flower essences consistently in my practice. It is difficult to explain or understand the workings of the flower essences until one has actually experienced them. The simplest explanation I can offer you is this:

I am the writer and the actor of my play (my reality; my life). When I am attached to an emotion, I cannot recognize the emotion. I am too busy acting it out. Flower essences allow me to move away from the center stage and into the balcony where I can now see clearly the role I have taken on in life and what I am creating. The more I see, the more I realize that I am responsible for my creations; my choices; my life. If I am not happy with my play, I am now free to rewrite it so I can act differently. This is what I call seeing through the eyes of truth instead of the eyes of the emotion. Flower essences are the doorways that allow me to see truthfully.

Flower essences take us directly to the eyes of truth. They help us vibrate to a higher level of consciousness. Much like an electrical charge from an outlet, flower essences charge our electrical system into high gear. They empower us to see, feel and experience life in different ways and at different vibrations.

Our thoughts, our words and our actions are our creative forces. Flower essences allow us to hear our thoughts and words clearly and be accountable for our actions. They put the responsibility for our actions right where it belongs, with the individual.

What flower essences will NOT do is make choices for us. We are the creators of our world. We are given free will so we can create anything we choose. We are free to change our choices; we are also free to continue our old patterns of behavior.

Not everyone wants to see the truth; the truth often brings us to a painful place that we have denied or pretended did not exist. It is easy to avoid this pain if we spend our time blaming and resenting everyone and everything that we have surrounded ourselves with in life. However, that will not heal us. It will only keep us in unhealthy patterns of behaviors. The flower essences allowed me to see clearly my unhealthy behaviors. I was then able to use the flower essences to help Joshua see his.

Facing the Pains of Our Past

Flower essences take us right to the doorway of the pain we have been hiding in our bodies. These are the same doorways we have forced shut; the same doorways we run from. To heal we must stop running and hiding; we must begin dealing.

As we go through layers of healing, we are able to move away from the pain. First we must recognize it; honor it and finally forgive it. These three steps release us from the pains of our past so they no longer hold power over us.

Joshua and I faced our pains together. With the help of flower essences we learned that we had to stop the patterns of fear and frustration that had turned into blame and resentment. This shift of energy did not come easily, it took time and energy. Although novices to emotional healing practices, we were willing participants.

As I learned more about vibration medicines and spiritual healing, I helped Joshua work through each layer. Always at the end of each layer, he was met by fear. Fear was and still is his resistance factor. Fear protected him for many years; it would not easily be dismissed. As he learned to look within, he recognized the aspects of himself that kept him in a cycle of self abuse by coming face to face with his fear. He did not always like what he saw, but he honored it as a part of who he had become, certain he was ready and willing to change it.

Recognizing our patterns is the beginning of our ability to change our "self." Becoming conscious of his patterns, Joshua could now work to change them, one pattern at a time. It took years for Joshua to rise to a greater consciousness and to finally come to a greater understanding of peace. Healing is a lifelong journey. Each step Joshua took to maintain his sense of truth, compassion and understanding, the greater his ability to lessen the symptoms that plagued him for years.

Will Joshua always be a sensitive being? Absolutely! He came that way so he could teach the severity of chemical poisoning. He continues to honor the importance of maintaining a pure state for his body, mind, and soul. Why would he want to be anything else?

Does his body have to react violently? Absolutely not! Joshua learned to listen to his body with subtle energies of communication by mastering the art of healing.

Today, when one of my children creates an illness within themselves, I immediately receive a phone call with one question: "What am I doing to create this?" Muscle testing allows me to help them see where they have hidden their emotion and to understand the language of their symptoms. Once they take responsibility for their illness (pains), they can consciously shift the energy by changing their behaviors through their thoughts, words and actions. It is this shift in energy that allows the body to heal.

The emotion that shows itself as a physical symptom, be it pain, rash, or infection, is demanding attention through the only means it knows how, the physical body. It will move with nothing less than love and forgiveness.

Frustration Turned to Compassion

Watching Joshua heal was always an educational experience. From elementary school through college, he was my thesis. I was receiving my education in healing as he received his Master's in Public Policy. He taught through the language of his body; I learned what his body was teaching. It was a partnership made in heaven. Of that I have no doubt.

I will admit that some lessons were more challenging than others. His high school years were the most challenging which made my attention to details paramount. During our ongoing battles with the administration, I had a moment of realization that was undeniable--

emotions create physical symptoms. The flower essences helped me see this moment clearly.

In elementary and middle school, Joshua's concerns were being honored; his voice was being heard. Solutions were found and Joshua moved beyond the fear and frustration. However, high school was an entirely different experience. Joshua was not honored; he was barely heard.

During his high school years, Joshua feared he would not be able to go to school and then became frustrated because no one seemed to care. These two energies created an inner state of turmoil. Fear and frustration prevented his organs from flushing toxins through his system. The more he allowed these emotions to rule his life, the more sensitive he became. There was a time when even a minute dose of a chemical created an instant reaction; from there, more fear and frustration, more chemical reactions.

Unhealthy emotions had become part of his daily routine. His body was responding to the emotions he was feeding it, and none of it was nurturing. His fears and frustrations escalated to the point that he was now consumed by them.

It is one thing to have a moment of fear and frustration; it is another to live in it day and night. Fear and frustration had become him. I was certain that his emotions intensified his reactions. To make matters worse, my own fears and frustrations were feeding into his. It was time for me to be accountable as well.

Over time, fear and frustration turned into resentment and blame. Joshua was now directing this energy outwardly toward others. I was doing the same. I understood why this was happening; no one was listening! As unhealthy as that was, what we were doing was equally unhealthy. I had to help him recognize his behaviors and then help him stop repeating them. First I had to stop myself.

It was confusing at first. What is a person to do who is constantly being denied the freedom to go to school? Isn't fear and frustration part of the natural progression of order? I had to start thinking outside the box; in other words, beyond how we are taught to behave under certain circumstances and situations.

No matter how pure the food and water, toxic thoughts and feelings interrupted his ability to heal, not to mention toxic chemicals. His mind and body were on a path of self destruction. I needed to help him hit the brakes. Joshua was about to learn accountability.

Coming to Peace

Unhealthy energy shared among the whole will not heal any thing or any one. Joshua and I were in a state of war and what we desired was peace. We lost sight of the mission. It was time to refocus.

I now understood that if Joshua were to heal, he had to stop directing this unhealthy energy outwardly as resentment and blame. This was a waste of energy. Why? Because he could not heal others; he could only heal himself. We had forgotten our greatest lesson: *healing occurs within.*

Those were powerful words and I understood their meaning. As long as we blame and resent out there, we can never heal in here, within our "self." Were we ready to honor these words by redirecting our energy back to where it belonged? Were we ready to honor our emotions so we could begin to change our "self" into the person we wanted to be as opposed to the person we had now become?

"Josh, it is time for both of us to come to peace with the situation we have created. I don't want to win the war. I don't even know how we got to war. What I want is for you to be at peace, at home and at school."

This was the conversation we had the night before he spoke to the school board members. I was a counselor and I had forgotten that which I was teaching others. Truth is not angry or hateful; truth is not fearful or guilty. Truth is truth. What I also knew from my prior experience is that truth equals love; these two energies are of the same vibration. If we wanted our outcome to be surrounded by love, we had to start speaking in truth.

"Let's leave our frustrations and fears at home. Let's go to the school board meeting and speak the truth and see where truth takes us."

After hearing these words, Joshua felt better about what he had to do. The one thing he knew about himself was that truth came easily through his words. Anything else made him ill.

When he entered the school board meeting that night, he did so free of fear and frustration. He did what I asked; he left them both at home. He brought a light to that room that began a shift in energy. We had a long way to go, but the process had begun. Love and forgiveness replaced fear and frustration. We welcomed them in; would we be able to keep them on board?

These new energies felt good to Joshua. I enjoyed watching him change. Instead of being angry toward those in power; he practiced feeling sad for them. After all, they could not have known what they were doing. A healthy educator would never deny a child his right to an education. Joshua was beginning to understand that those in power were as fearful and frustrated as he was. We were all sharing the same energy in different ways. Instead of wasting his energy trying to change them, Joshua chose to change him "self."

Much like a chess game, Joshua made the first move. He consciously chose to move pieces of himself toward forgiveness, and the energy that once consumed him began to shift. It shifted in a different direction to open new doorways and new possibilities.

Stepping into a new doorway can happen in a moment or it can take time and patience. This type of healing was new to us. It took time for us to recreate. Often fear and frustration wanted to bring us back to war. Sometimes we picked up our swords and joined them. As my knowledge and skill with the flower essences expanded, we were always reminded that war was not the way to peace. Together we practiced forgiveness and understanding. We remembered to be compassionate. We learned the way of truth.

Our practice of avoiding fear and frustration did not deter our mission in any way. Our conscious use of other forces moved it in the direction we intended from the beginning. Our mission was now on track to create a healthy environment in which all children could learn and play. Truth brought us there in a very gentle, peaceful way. The flower essences helped us see the light at the end of the tunnel.

Emotional Storage Tanks

Years have passed, and the flower essences have taught me a great deal more than I could have imagined. I watched the language of the physical body, and I can assure you it is a language in need of attention. Each physical symptom is the spirit's way of speaking to us. The language is very clear, "Pay attention to me, I am not feeling loved."

Emotions are a flow of continuous energy much like the tides, moving through the water within our bodies. If we sit in an emotion for more than the time needed to move to a greater understanding of one's self, the energy of that particular emotion will find its way into the appropriate body part (or as I call it, storage tank) waiting for us to recognize it for what it is: a distortion of love that begins with "fear of not being loved."

Whatever we uncover as we begin to heal, whether it is guilt or shame, resentment or blame, frustration or disappointment, the underlying energy waiting to be discovered will ALWAYS bring us back to "fear of not being loved."

This is the beauty of understanding spiritual healing. I either heal or I don't by the choices I make to love myself or deny myself love. We are constantly being challenged to bring ourselves back to a state of loving one's self.

By recognizing the physical symptom and the body part being affected, I am able to understand the language of the body. Joshua's body had a clear language that needed interpretation. I became the interpreter until he learned to understand it himself.

We are all patterning beings and Joshua had a clear pattern. He overused and over-abused two organs that stored the bulk of his emotions, his liver and his gall bladder; both organs are housed in the *third chakra*.

Healing the Liver & Gall Bladder

Of my three children, Joshua was more sensitive than his two sisters. There was a reason for his sensitivities; frustration and fear were the principal factors.

The liver is a vital organ with a wide range of functions, including detoxification. Frustration is the emotion that is stored in the liver. Joshua was often frustrated with his inability to be like other children. He wanted to be "normal," free of the limitations chemical sensitivities demanded of him.

Because his liver was clogged with frustration, chemicals seriously aggravated his system; however, it was Joshua's fears and frustrations that caused his extreme sensitivities. Joshua had to change his behaviors by being responsible for his actions and allowing the school board to be responsible for theirs.

Frustration would not take him where he wanted to go. If he wanted to be healthy, he had to change his frustrating thoughts into forgiving thoughts. Through forgiveness, he could let go of the anger he felt toward those who denied his right to be at school.

Forgiveness also helped him to love all of himself, even the sensitive being he came to be. Joshua finally came to peace with his differences which helped him see that he was as normal as any other child.

Forgiveness turned his frustrations into love and his symptoms lessened in severity. Did they go away completely? No, because our bodies will ALWAYS respond when they are being poisoned. Joshua's body was a great communicator and Joshua learned to be a great listener.

The gall bladder was the other organ that played havoc with Joshua's system. The gall bladder aids in fat digestion and holds the emotion of fear. Joshua's gall bladder was always filled with fear, which hampered his ability to break down fats especially those that are not easily digestible. Cow dairy is a fat that is not easy to digest. This caused his sensitivity to cow dairy products.

When Joshua felt safe and secure at home and at school, his gall bladder could function properly. To get to those feelings of safety and security, he had to face his fears by expressing his truth to those in authority, and continue to do so with the hope of having his needs met. He did so gracefully.

A vegetarian diet was Joshua's healthiest choice, and to this day he will tell me that the meal that suits his digestion best is a piece of whole grain bread with beans, olive oil and goat cheese; add organic arugula to that mix and I have one happy boy!

There is so much that I have learned about the path to healing. It is a complex lesson that Joshua easily taught. Healthy food, pure water and a clean environment begin to heal the physical body. The ability to express one's thoughts and feelings through forgiveness and compassion completes the process. The combination of both forces nurtures a healthy mind and body followed by a happy life. Once he turned this corner, Joshua learned the power of loving the spiritual being he came to be.

Joshua's Favorite Flowers

Throughout his life, Joshua collected layers of fears and frustration. To heal he had to unravel what his fears and frustrations were attached to. Each layer revealed more of the same old patterns that were in need of change. He could no longer deny his attachment to these energies.

Eventually, the unraveling brought him back to the source: *fear of not being loved.*

Joshua had to learn how to love all of who he came to be. The flower essences were a means to that end, helping him to recognize how his choices that led to fear and frustration affected his health.

Larch was the flower essence he used most often to help recognize the fears that now consumed him. Larch enabled him to come face to face with his fears especially those that were attached to fear of failures and fear to make mistakes. Larch did not heal these energies for him; it simply allowed him to recognize them, and with recognition comes the opportunity to change.

There were many other flowers that helped Joshua see through the eyes of his truth. These are the ones that Joshua often used to help him come to peace.

- Larch helped Joshua recognize his fears of failure, insecurity, and rejection, allowing him to feel secure in his own decisions and to have compassion for those who refused to understand.
- Cerato helped him recognize the decisions that made him most happy and allowed him to stand strong in his beliefs.
- Mimulus helped him recognize the original fear that always begins the process. As with every original fear, Joshua was afraid of not being loved and revealed itself through the physical body as digestive issues and sensitivities.
- Willow helped him see that frustration and resentment were a part of his illness. Willow helped begin the process of forgiving everything and everyone he blamed and resented for causing his pain including himself.

Healing is an on-going process, and Joshua continues to heal today. His sensitivity levels have diminished significantly over time. The more he focuses his energy on what he loves in life, the happier his body responds. He continues to be responsible for his health by the choices he makes. He loves fresh organic food and drinks only pure water. His body still speaks clearly if and when he is being poisoned by his surroundings.

The difference today is that he understands what he has to do to remain healthy. He uses his energy to create a world that is as free of chemicals as possible. He recognizes when his fears and frustrations surface and honors them for the opportunity to change. He remembers to balance himself by focusing on the joy in his life; and there are many of those to focus upon.

Today, Joshua is following the divine mission he came to do. His Master's degree in public policy has created a position that inspires many leaders to seek out his counsel and advice. Joshua willingly shares his truth with others.

Chapter Twelve

~ Spiritual Contracts ~

Thirty years have passed since Joshua's birth. Each time we reach a higher level of healing, there is more to learn. Recently, with the help of flower essences, I have been observing seven distinct personality types that are interconnected to the seven spiritual chakras.

I recognized these personality types by observing how my family and clients consistently created the same physical symptoms in the same general areas of the body. There was a clear pattern developing, and I was consciously watching it evolve.

The spiritual body was sending signals through the physical body; signals that we refer to as symptoms. Each signal or symptom is a spiritual attempt to guide us back to our true nature, our true "self," an attempt to move away from pain and back toward love. What we have forgotten is that love is not painful.

The physical body is our spiritual guidance system, and a symptom of the physical body is nothing more than a language that says, "Hey, you have strayed from your divine path; turn around!" EVERY physical symptom we experience is an opportunity to make a different choice. It is easy to follow divine guidance if we listen to the signals being emitted through our physical body.

The signal may begin as a twitch, an ache or a small rash. If we continue to move away from our truth or our divine path, the signal will intensify trying to force our attention. If we continue to deny further, the signal will scream and disease may be the end result. A disease is often the only indicator that clearly gets our attention and stops us from going any further. Healing could be less complicated if we learn to change our patterns of behavior when our signals are subtle.

It would seem that changing a pattern of behavior could be effortless; recognize the pattern and change it. Truthfully, however, it is one of the most difficult challenges we face as humans. Self destructive or self defeating behaviors are often the path we are programmed to follow; hating our jobs, our lives, our choices and feeling we are powerless to change any of them. These feelings keep us from love.

The truth is we are free to change our job, our life and our choice in any moment. We are not powerless to change our "self;" we are choosing not to change for various reasons. These reasons become our excuses and explanations; ego tactics that keep us from sharing our love with others.

The longer we continue to deny our truth, the more chaotic and dramatic our lives become until one day, universal energy may force our hand. This may happen through the loss of a job, a disease, a divorce or a death. As time goes on, we may realize that it is this life altering event that forced us to turn around from the direction we were heading and begin to heal our "self."

My own healing practice has taught me that it is much less painful to change my direction with the more subtle signals; the twitch, the ache or the small rash. By making a different choice in the moment I am directed, I am able to avoid the more serious side effects caused by denying my spiritual signals.

As this information was revealed, a whole new set of questions were in need of answers.

- What if we are *divinely designed* to vibrate to a higher state of spiritual understanding of our "self?"
- What if we are connected to a *collective contract* that states, "I choose to be born to help create peace on Earth?"
- What if we also have an *individual contract* that states, "I will help create peace on Earth by creating peace within myself and then I will help create peace within my family?"

− What if we are given all the tools necessary to create that peace?

− What if we have forgotten and it is now time to remember?

I believe that everyone who enters the Earth plane is bound by two contracts: an individual and a collective contract. One has a direct effect upon the other. Both are initiated for one divine purpose: *To help create peace on Earth.* If you are here, you have spiritually signed these two contracts; and if you are reading *Joshua's Lessons*, it is time for you to remember the peaceful person you came to be.

The Individual & Collective Contracts

The individual contract clearly states that I will help create peace on Earth the only way possible--by creating peace within myself. This process begins with the individual's willingness to remember that every thought is an opportunity to choose peace above all else. The power to change angry thoughts into peaceful thoughts directs our energy towards a peaceful outcome.

Spiritual healing takes place through the vibration of peace. Peace is an intimate experience. Although we are designed to love this aspect, we are similarly taught to fear it. Sadly, fear often takes precedence over love, which is why it was so important for Joshua to love every aspect of himself, including his sensitive nature. As long as he feared being different, he could never come to peace with himself and he could never heal. Loving his differences would bring him to peace.

Separateness is also a part of spiritual healing. To create healthy interconnectedness (relationships) we must first experience separateness. Separateness allows us to see our differences, our individuality. As we learn who we are individually, we are then able to share our true self with the whole. It is a powerful moment in healing when we realize that we must experience separateness to be whole, and at the same time we are not separate from the whole.

Maintaining individuality among a group can be challenging. Group energy is very powerful. We are easily drawn into the thoughts and beliefs of those around us. We easily mold ourselves to meet the needs of others, while denying our own needs. To enter the vibration of love toward peace, we must separate from other's beliefs. We must begin to recognize what feels true to one's self. Recognizing our feelings and expressing our feelings allows us the opportunity to meet our individual needs, separating our 'self' from what is expected. Watching Joshua voice his needs to those in authority was a powerful lesson for everyone in the community. Choosing to leave school to meet his individual need was his moment of truth and truth leads to peace.

The individual contract binds us to a collective contract, our interconnectedness to one another and to the divine source. As we create peace within the self, we are charged to help create peace within the family. The only way to help others come to peace is to come to peace with one's self; and the way to peace is ALWAYS through compassion understanding, which then directs us toward love. Every choice we make has a direct affect upon the people we are surrounded by, especially those we love the most. Choosing love above all else allows us to share that love with family and friends.

To complete his divine mission, Joshua had to take responsibility for his thoughts, words and actions. His angry thoughts prompted angry words that had the potential to create an angry outcome. Peaceful thoughts, on the other hand, prompted peaceful words and had the potential to create a peaceful outcome. To find his way toward peace, Joshua had to recognize those aspects that kept him in a cycle of turmoil and pain. Only then could he remember that he had the power to change himself, one thought at a time.

Healing takes on a whole new meaning when we come to understand that, "I am my thoughts, and my words create my reality." We begin to heal when we learn to master our 'self' through our thoughts, words and actions. For Joshua to heal, he would have to remember who he came to be and how he wanted to share that identity with others. His remembering took him right to his *third chakra*.

Mastering the Third Chakra

The seven spiritual chakras are connected to the physical body through the organs, glands and systems of the body. As part of our individual contract, we are required to choose one of these chakras with which we will come to Earth to learn our individual lessons. These are the lessons we must *master* in this lifetime. Our individual chakra will help guide us toward our divine path by speaking clearly to us through our physical and emotional symptoms.

This is a story in itself and one I will be more than happy to share with you at a future time. For the sake of our story right now, however, it is important to focus our attention on the third chakra personality because I believe, like Joshua, our highly sensitively children come to Earth to heal through the energy of the third chakra; the one we call the solar plexus.

As I watched Joshua heal, I began to take note of other sensitive children that asked for help in healing. Many had the same imbalances as Joshua, both physically and emotionally. Many were auditory learners. This alignment of energies brought me to a new understanding of sensitive children and their connection to the third chakra.

The third chakra houses the *gall bladder, liver, stomach, pancreas, adrenal glands and digestive system.* When out of balance, the third chakra personalities are fear addicts. The fears they are most connected to are *fear of failure, fear to make a mistake, fear of the wrong decision and fear of rejection.* These types of fears are stored in the gall bladder.

Any one of these fears has the potential to manifest in the physical body as digestive disorders. The gall bladder is often affected first, and the physical symptoms may appear as *bloating, burping, gas, reflux, lower back pain and dairy allergies.*

It is essential for this personality type to avoid foods that aggravate the gall bladder including *fried food, hydrogenated oils, pork and all cow dairy products.* Along with digestive problems, cow dairy can cause mucus membrane problems for this personality type.

When angry they are more apt to become frustrated with their inability to make a good decision. They are less apt to resent or blame others. Frustration with one self is stored in the liver as anger. An imbalance in the liver can manifest in the physical body as *pains, skin rashes, infections, inability to focus and chemical sensitivities.*

As Joshua began to heal, he recognized that chemicals had a profound effect on his ability to learn and focus, even more so when he became frustrated. When his liver was unable to perform its functions, his body often used his skin to flush chemicals quickly through his system; hives, rashes and boils were a quick fix to a serious problem. A clogged liver is better able to heal by avoiding the things that aggravate it including *city water, artificial ingredients, artificial sweeteners, preservatives and environmental chemicals.*

Dairy allergies and chemical sensitivities are common with this personality type because most of their emotional energy is stored in their digestive system. The more fearful and frustrated they become, the more sensitive their body responds. The third chakra personality will heal their fears and frustrations by understanding and accepting their sensitive nature.

When in balance the third chakra personalities are the decision makers of the world. They are healthy when they are decisive and confident. Their spiritual path is connected to learning how to make good decisions early in life so they are prepared for their divine mission later in life. Hence, this personality type loves to learn. They cannot get enough input. The more they know, the more capable they are at making good decisions which in turn helps to alleviate their fears.

The third chakra personality is charged with mastering the vibration of certainty. To get there, they must move through their fears. Healing took a huge step when Joshua finally agreed to speak before the school board. This was his moment of truth; the moment he came face to face with his fears.

The third chakra personality will be called upon throughout their lives to make decisions; certainty must become them. Arrogance and superiority have no place in their healing process, although they will often revert to both as a means to hide their own inferiorities. Neither will serve their mission.

There is great importance to this charge. As they mature the third chakra personality will take on the responsibility of representing those who are less fortunate or unable to represent themselves. They become the leaders and decision makers of the world; their divine mission is to lead through truth. Anything else will make them ill.

They are guided toward positions where their decisions have the potential to affect many individuals: *CEOs of companies, lawyers, judges, coaches and politicians.* It made sense to me that they would come as auditory learners. To make good decisions for others, they must first be good listeners.

Joshua's ability to maintain a healthy gall bladder and liver was essential. He learned to recognize his fears and frustrations so he could begin to change his patterns of behavior. He avoided the chemicals that aggravated his third chakra. These were the secrets to healing his allergies and sensitivities. I cannot stress enough the importance of pure water, organic food and a chemical free environment for this personality type. Because of the changes we made, Joshua is healthy today.

Joshua had an innate sense of knowing this charge from a very early age. I had an innate sense of understanding that he picked me as his mother to help him master his third chakra vibration. Together, ours was a divine mission.

One Last Story

"Mom, I can't think; I can't focus. I have this paper due and I need your help!" The year was 2009 and Joshua was studying for his Master's Degree in Public Policy. He was no longer a child; he was a man. However, in that moment, he was my little boy again needing my counsel.

I recognized these words from his childhood which he often expressed when a chemical had poisoned his liver. Lack of focus and concentration was evident long before a physical symptom manifested in his body. Those words instantly brought me back to the memory when the water he was drinking at the school bubbler made him angry and ill.

My response was instantaneous. "What have you been drinking?" Just like old times, Joshua had an issue, I had a question.

"Oh...." I could hear his mind trailing off into the near distant past. "I got sick of buying bottled water so I put an expensive water system on my tap. I've been drinking from that system lately."

The words of long ago spewed from my mouth, "Don't drink the water!" Joshua tried desperately to assure me the filter was top quality.

"It has to work!" I could feel his old frustrations popping up. He spent a lot of money on that water filter and did not want to admit it could be the problem.

"Josh, stop the water for a little while and see if it helps. It's the only way to know for sure, and take some dandelion root to help your body move the chemical out of your liver."

I did not hear from him for quite a few days and thought I would call to check on his status. The voice on the other end of the phone assured me he was healthy again "You were right, Mom. It was the water." A lesson Joshua needed to remember: Pure water is his very best friend; his body and mind will allow nothing else.

Epilogue by Joshua Wojcik

You've just finished reading about my childhood through my mother's recollections. Now, 29 years old and mostly free of the symptoms of chemical sensitivities, I've had time to reflect and feel I can share a different perspective growing up with chemical sensitivities.

First, let me say, I wouldn't trade my experiences for a "normal" life. Although difficult to deal with at times, my chemical sensitivities have given me a heightened awareness of the foods I eat, the water I drink and of my daily surroundings.

During my childhood and teen years I had to continuously explain why I couldn't partake in birthday cake at my playmates' parties and had to kindly decline to join friends at the local Chinese restaurant. I'm not sure if I can confidently say that I felt the same way as a kid, but now I believe being chemically sensitive allowed me to develop a strong self discipline and a willingness to be different; more importantly to celebrate that difference.

Now that I'm older, I'm proud that I was allergic to all types of carcinogens, artificial additives and the like. These things aren't good for anyone. It just turned out that my body rejected them immediately which I now find amazing.

Today, I still eat all natural foods, use all natural cleaners and try to keep my environment as chemical free as possible. Luckily my wife has completely adopted my natural lifestyle. She knows the foods I can and cannot eat, the cleaners that are safe to use, and the items never to bring into our home. When we first lived together, I had to ask her to ditch all her beloved scented candles; she understood and begrudgingly threw them away.

There are still incidences of course. I recently tried to switch from bottled spring water to filtered city water, liking the idea of supporting local water resources. Unfortunately, my body still cannot handle the chlorine and fluoride additives. After a month or two, finding my body literally shaking, my digestion compromised and unable to concentrate long enough to read a paragraph in a book, I gave up and went back to spring water.

Similarly, lawn pesticides still do a number on me. I live in a condo that sprays once a month. Every time, without fail, I wake up the next morning with red irritated eyes, feeling groggy with low back pains as my body tries to detoxify the chemicals. I've been having a bit of a tug of war with the condo association over this; some things never change.

It's been a decade since I've experienced any severe allergic reactions. Today my day to day life is pretty run of the mill; however, I still remember what it was like to go through days fearing some incidental contact with one chemical or another. I think that was often the hardest part. It's difficult to go through each day not knowing if you'll unwittingly run into a chemical that will result in a restless night of hives or a morning of swollen glands and a pounding headache. The constant worry can be exhausting in and of itself.

One of the most important lessons I learned through my experience is that the constant worrying over the next allergic reaction only held me back. In the end my family and I took necessary precautions. We tried to change my daily environment both at home and at school; however, we couldn't prevent everything. Both my mom and I had to come to grips with that. There were going to be some days of sickness and getting angry only made life more stressful.

Luckily, most people in my life were very supportive which helped make life a lot easier. Friends were always on the lookout, "oh boy don't smell that Woj, that could kill ya." They modified their behavior for my benefit and often warned me of nearby perfumes or chemicals so I could remove myself from the situation.

Working my way through my pre-teen and teen years required a willingness to inform people about my allergies and ask the school to accommodate my needs. Eventually I tried to avoid getting too worked up about the whole thing.

Living with chemical sensitivities required a fulltime awareness of my surroundings, but it never prevented me from having a childhood full of wonderful experiences and fond memories. Thanks to the many supportive people in my life, especially my mom who was my tireless advocate, I had a great childhood. Together we were able to create a safe place for me to live, learn and play and initiated changes that benefited everyone.

Joshua Wojcik

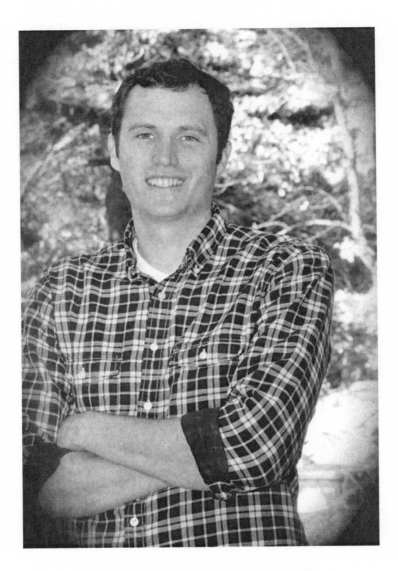

Joshua...at peace with himself...

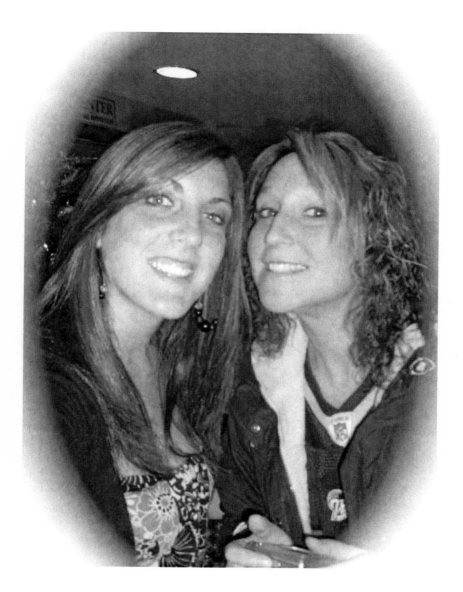

Holly Beth & Shannon
together you are a light to the world!

Resources

Linda Wojcik, BFP
Nutritional Kinesiologist--Spiritual Intuitive
North Stonington CT
www.healingyou.com

William Shevin, MD, D.Ht.
Woodstock CT
www.drshevin.com

Bach® Flower Remedies
www.bachflower.com

CT Northeast Organic Farming Association
www.ctnofa.org

Everybody's Guide to Homeopathic Medicines
By Stephen Cummings, MD & Dana Ullman, MPH

The Homeopathy Bible
By Ambika Wauters

Foods that Heal
By Dr. Bernard Jensen